Manual of Child Neurology:
Problem Based Approach to Common Disorders

Authored By

Mohammed M. S. Jan

Professor & Consultant of Pediatric Neurology
Department of Pediatrics, Faculty of Medicine, King Abdulaziz
University
Jeddah
Kingdom of Saudi Arabia

CONTENTS

About the Author   *i*

Foreword   *ii*

Preface   *iii*

Acknowledgement   *iv*

CHAPTERS

1.   History Taking   3

2.   Neurological Examination   6

3.   Examining the Difficult Child   14

4.   Normal Development   17

5.   Developmental Disorders   21

6.   Cerebral Palsy   27

7.   Neurodegenerative Disorders   35

8.   Neurometabolic Disorders   42

9.   Seizures and Epilepsy   47

10. Seizure Semiology   62

11. Febrile Seizures   72

12. Meningitis & Encephalitis   78

13. Infant Hypotonia   83

14. Muscle Weakness   87

15. Acute Hemiplegia   90

16. Abnormal Movements   94

17. Unsteady Gait   98

18. Headache & Migraine   105

19. Demyelinating Disorders   111

20. DNR Decisions   116

21. Brain Death Criteria   123

22. Communicating Bad News   129

     Index   134

ABOUT THE AUTHOR

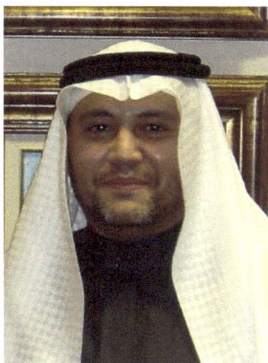

This eBook was written and edited by Mohammed M. S. Jan, who is a Professor and Consultant of Pediatric Neurology and Clinical Neurophysiology, Department of Pediatrics, Faculty of Medicine, King Abdulaziz University, Jeddah, Kingdom of Saudi Arabia. Prof. Jan was born and raised in Makkah, Saudi Arabia. He graduated from the Faculty of Medicine, king Abdulaziz University in Jeddah with an excellent grade (honor degree). He received post-graduate training from 1991 to 1998 at Dalhousie University, Halifax, Nova Scotia, Canada.

Prof. Jan obtained several certificates including the American Board of Pediatrics, Fellowship of the Royal College of Physicians of Canada (FRCPC) in Pediatrics, FRCPC in Neurology, EMG Certification, and EEG Certification by the Canadian Society of Clinical Neurophysiologists. He has more than 80 publications in peer reviewed national and international journals. Currently, Prof. Jan is an active member of several national and international organizations including the Saudi Chapter of Epilepsy, Pan Arab Child Neurology Association, the American Epilepsy Society, the International Child Neurology Association, and the Canadian Society of Child Neurology. He also serves on several editorial and review boards of several national and international journals. Prof. Jan received several awards including 2 Merit awards presented by the Saudi Council in Canada for academic achievements, Post-doctoral Research Award presented by the British Council, 2 Recognition Award presented by the Faculty of Medicine, and 3 Research Excellence award presented by the Deanship of Scientific Research, King Abdulaziz University.

Finally, the author would like to thank his parents, wife, and four sons for their ongoing support and love. He dedicates this eBook to all medical students and pediatric residents and hopes that the manual provides a simple and practical introduction to Pediatric Neurology.

Jeddah
Saudi Arabia

FOREWORD

This eBook was written and edited by Prof. Mohammed M. S. Jan with an aim to present a simplified, organized, and comprehensive problem based approach to common pediatric neurological disorders directed to the level of medical students, pediatric and neurology residents, general practitioners and general pediatricians. It is composed of 22 chapters with many tabled and illustrated figures and photos. This eBook will provide a concise outline with practical tips to facilitate proper diagnosis and management of various neurological disorders.

Prof. Ali O. Saabat
Faculty of Medicine
King Abdulaziz University
Jeddah
Saudi Arabia

PREFACE

Pediatric neurology is considered a relatively new and evolving subspecialty. Over the last century, remarkable advances at both the basic and clinical levels have considerably improved our ability to evaluate and treat children with neurological disorders. These disorders are common and many cases seen by general pediatricians are primarily neurological accounting for up to 30% of all consultations to pediatrics with a high ratio of follow-up visits to new patients of about 3:1. Many medical students feel that their teaching experiences in neurology are not strong and only a small percentage actually select pediatric neurology as the first future career choice. This is not encouraging given the strong demand for this specialty in our region. Apart from large textbooks, limited pediatric neurology references are available for medical students and pediatric residents. It was for this reason that this manual was developed. In our experience, many of undergraduate medical students refer to deficient and oversimplified references that do not enable them to deal with pediatric neurology patients adequately.

Please note that no financial contributions or any potential conflict of interest to any of the eBook chapters exist.

Mohammed M. S. Jan
Professor & Consultant of Pediatric Neurology
Department of Pediatrics
Faculty of Medicine
King Abdulaziz University
Jeddah
Kingdom of Saudi Arabia
E-mail: mmsjan@yahoo.ca

iv

ACKNOWLEDGEMENT

The author would like to extend the warmest thanks and gratitude to **King Abdulaziz University** for the valuable support and guidance.

CHAPTER 1

History Taking

Abstract: Careful and detailed history is the key to accurate diagnosis. Children with neurological disorders may have long clinical course, multiple symptoms, and complicated histories. Therefore, an organized approach to history taking is required. It is a good practice to keep a problem list that would prioritize various manifestation and complications. Disorders that are inactive or remote should be lower on the list. This chapter deals with the organization and important details in the history taking of children with neurological complaints. History of the most commonly encountered disorders, such as developmental delay, epilepsy, and cerebral palsy, is described in details in the designated chapters.

Keywords: Neurological, History taking, Presenting illness, Problem list, System review, Development, Past medical/Family history, Social history.

PROBLEM LIST

During the process of history taking, various problems should be identified and organized in a problem list. For example, a child with cerebral palsy may have epilepsy, feeding difficulties, recurrent chest infections, and constipation. In complicated and chronic patients, the physician may not have enough time in one visit to address all issues. This is understandable and several visits and consultations may be needed to address all issues. However, the physician should identify these problems and prioritize them. In busy practice or student exams one should focus on the active and more serious complaints.

HISTORY OF PRESENTING ILLNESS

The parent's words should be used. Diagnostic labels should not be taken for granted, as misdiagnosis is not uncommon. This is particularly true for cerebral palsy and epilepsy. We frequently encounter children diagnosed with cerebral palsy who end up having a progressive CNS disorder and patients with non-epileptic events diagnosed as epilepsy. The nature of the neurological manifestations should be clarified. The distinction between static (non-progressive) and progressive clinical course is very important. In patients with seizures, careful and detailed event description is the cornerstone of an accurate diagnosis. A timed description of the child's behavior during the event is needed for accurate classification and localization. The physician should remember to include the child in the conversation who may provide valuable information. If the description is not clear, the physician can ask the parent to mimic the event. The history of each event should be divided in four stages including preictal, beginning of the seizure, ictal, and postictal phase. This ordered approach is recommended for any paroxysmal events, including recurrent headaches. In the preictal phase, provoking or precipitating factors should be sought of such as fever, illness, ingestion, compliance, and head injury. The time of the seizure is important as some occur predominantly in sleep (benign rolandic seizures, tonic seizures, and frontal lobe seizures). History of any brief focal signs or symptoms (aura) at the beginning of the more dramatic seizure should be obtained. Anxious parents tend to describe the most dramatic part of the seizure and ignore the more subtle initial focal symptoms. Tonic seizures immediately preceded by crying or minor trauma should alert the physician to the diagnosis of breath-holding spells. Falls following standing in a stressful situation (classroom) and preceded by dizziness suggests vasovagal syncope. During the seizure, the exact description of the clinical manifestations and their duration is needed. Clusters of tonic spasms upon awakening suggest infantile spasms. Postictal unilateral headache or transient weakness (Todd's paresis) has a lateralizing value indicating a contralateral hemispheric origin. Postictal aphasia (inability to talk despite being able to follow simple commands) suggests a seizure originating from the speech area of the dominant hemisphere. Visual field defects have localizing value indicating occipital lobe origin.

SYSTEM REVIEW

Many common neurological disorders, such as cerebral palsy, affect multiple organs and systems. Detailed system review is needed to identify important associated manifestations or complications of the underlying

CNS disease. Common examples include feeding difficulties, vomiting, constipation, recurrent chest infections, incontinence, and recurrent urinary tract infections. If the child has a single problem, such as seizures, then detailed system review becomes a lower priority.

DEVELOPMENTAL HISTORY

Detailed developmental history is needed. The nature of the neurological manifestations should be clarified. The distinction between static (non-progressive) and progressive clinical course is very important. Classically, loss of previously acquired milestones (regression) marks the onset of most neurodegenerative disorders with subsequent progressive neurological deterioration. However, some degenrative or metabolic disorders have a slow rate of progression and can be misdiagnosed as cerebral palsy. Therefore, clear developmental regression may not be evident, particularly in the early stages of the disease or at a younger age of onset.

PAST MEDICAL HISTORY

Detailed prenatal, natal, and postnatal history is critical in order to identify risk factors or possible etiology of the child's neurological complaint. Examples include fetal movements (decreased in peripheral nervous disorders such as spinal muscular atrophy), maternal illness such as diabetes mellitus or hypertension, fetal distress, traumatic delivery, bleeding, infection, or jaundice. Beware of using the label "asphyxia" which does not equal fetal distress. Some asphyxiated babies are not distressed at birth and many distressed babies do not suffer from asphyxia. Findings suggestive of asphyxia include clinical neonatal hypoxic ischemic encephalopathy (lethargy, poor feeding, hypotonia, and seizures), fetal acidosis, and evidence of multi-organ involvement (liver, heart, and kidney). In children with epilepsy, enquiring about history of meningitis, encephalitis, head injury, and febrile seizures is mandatory.

DRUGS

Detailed drug history is important particularly in patients with epilepsy. Details regarding the preparation, dose, and timing are important. Asking about the shape and color of various tablets and bottles would be useful as some parents may not remember the exact names. Always instruct the parents to bring all drugs with them for their follow-up clinic visits. It is amazing how common are mistakes and misunderstanding in dosing. For example, valproic acid syrup is available in two concentrations (200mg/3. 5ml or 200mg/ml). It is obvious that such mistakes can be serious. List of the drugs that were tried in the past should be obtained, as well as, reasons for withdrawal (lack of efficacy, side effects…etc). All side effects and hypersensitivity reactions should be documented. Cross reactivity is known to occur with some antiepileptic drugs, such as phenytoin and carbamazepine.

FAMILY HISTORY

Detailed family history is important as many neurological disorders are genetic with various modes of inheritance. Positive family history of epilepsy or consanguinity should raise the suspicion of an inherited genetic epileptic disorder, such as benign rolandic epilepsy. Family history of neurological disorders and early or unexplained deaths may indicate an undiagnosed inherited metabolic or NDD.

SOCIAL HISTORY

There are many social factors that can lead to, complicates, or result from various neurological disorders. For example, divorce, neglect, abuse, social and emotional deprivation can affect normal development and behavior. Many children with chronic neurological disorders, such as cerebral palsy, may be complicated or worsened by parental neglect and poor compliance with physiotherapy for example. As well, such disorders would add physical, emotional, and financial burden to the families. Identifying these problems would prevent their adverse effects and improve patient care. Questioning about mobility, transport, and availability of home helpers is needed for better management of these families.

SUMMARY

Detailed and careful history remains the key to accurate diagnosis. Comprehensive outline of the various aspects of the history is important, however, formulating a problem list is critical in complicated patients with multiple problems. No history is complete without a detailed family and social histories.

BIBLIOGRAPHY

Jan MMS, Khalifa MA. Nervous System and Development. In: Alhowasi MN (ed). Manual of Clinical Pediatrics. 4th Edition, Medical Book House, Riyadh, Saudi Arabia, p130-176, 2007.

CHAPTER 2

Neurological Examination

Abstract: Diagnosing neurological disorders requires accurate assessment including detailed neurological examination, which is an important step in formulating differential diagnosis and guiding laboratory investigations. Certain problems frequently face the junior physician including organizing a complete examination in a short time period, and consistently eliciting neurological signs. Certainly, repeated examinations and experience play an important role; however, solid knowledge and use of proper techniques are crucial for eliciting and interpreting neurological signs. Confidence in performing the nervous system examination appears to be critical in the proper evaluation and management of patients with neurological disorders. The approach and styles of different neurologists may vary; however, consistency in conducting the examination is critical. In this chapter, an outline for the examination of the nervous system is presented. Various procedures and techniques of eliciting physical signs and possible pitfalls in the nervous system examination will also be discussed.

Keywords: Neurological, Examination, General, Anthropometric, Signs, Higher cortical, Cranial nerves, Motor, Sensory/Cerebellum.

ORGANIZATION OF THE NEUROLOGICAL EXAM

It is always said that organization is the key to success. If the examiner has a consistently organized approach to the nervous system examination, he or she will less likely miss important parts of the examination. When we ask many students or residents to examine the nervous system, they frequently proceed to higher cortical functions, motor, or cranial nerve examination. This is a common mistake, as the examiner should first assess aspects of the general examination of relevance to the nervous system before conducting the core exam. These areas include the vital signs, anthropometric measurements, and general examination.

PROPOSED ORDERED APPROACH

1. Vital signs (including supine and standing blood pressure)

2. Anthropometric measurements (plotted on percentile charts)

3. General examination (skin, skull, spine, dysmorphism, meningeal signs)

4. Mental status examination (mini-mental status examination)

5. Cranial nerves (I to XII)

6. Motor system (inspection, palpation, and percussion)

7. Cerebellar examination (including gait)

8. Sensory system (peripheral and cortical sensations)

VITAL SIGNS

Examination of the nervous system is never complete without taking the vital signs. High temperature or hypothermia, particularly in infants, may indicate an underlying CNS infection. Temperature instability could be a sign of brain stem dysfunction. Blood pressure should be measured in the supine and standing positions to assess postural drop as in patients with vaso-vagal syncope. In patients with disturbed level of consciousness or seizures, high blood pressure and bradycardia (Cushing reflex) indicate increased intracranial pressure (*e.g.* due to hemorrhage, edema, or a space occupying lesion). The respiratory pattern may also indicate CNS dysfunction. Cheyne-Stokes breathing (periodic breathing pattern in which phases of hyperpnea regularly alternate with apnea) usually indicates bihemispheric dysfunction. Central hyperventilation (sustained, rapid, and deep hyperpnea) is produced by lesions in the lower midbrain or upper pons. Apneustic breathing (prolonged pause at full inspiration) may occur after damage to the mid or lower pons. Cluster breathing (disordered sequence of breaths with irregular pauses) may result from damage to the lower pons or upper medulla. Finally, ataxic breathing (completely irregular pattern of breathing with random deep and shallow breaths) is usually due to a lesion in the central medulla.

ANTHROPOMETRIC MEASUREMENTS

Weight, height, and head circumference should be measured and plotted on age appropriate percentile charts. The distinction between large head (macrocephaly) and large brain (megalencephaly) is important. If megalencephaly is suspected the parent's head circumferences should also be measured as benign autosomal dominant megalencephaly is one of the commonest causes. Microcephaly usually suggests brain atrophy or dysgenesis, however, diffuse craniosynostosis should be considered if signs or symptoms of raised intracranial pressure are associated. Short and tall stature, as well as, under or overweight may be associated with certain disorders and syndromes that affect growth and have associated neurological features or complications. A summary of these disorders is shown in Table **1**.

Table 1: Examples of the CNS features of some disorders and syndromes associated with abnormal stature or abnormal body weight.

Abnormality	Syndromes or diseases	CNS features
Short stature	Hypothyroidism Turner's syndrome Cockayne syndrome De Lang syndrome	Mental retardation Hearing loss Peripheral neuropathy Microbrachycephaly
Tall stature	Fragile X syndrome Sotos syndrome Weaver syndrome Marfan syndrome	Mental retardation Macrocephaly Progressive spasticity Risk of embolic stroke
Underweight	Congenital Rubella Seckel syndrome Rubinstein Taybi syndrome Fetal Hydantoin syndrome	Mental retardation, deafness Microcephaly EEG abnormalities Mental retardation, strabismus
Overweight	Beckwith Weidemann Bardet Biedl syndrome Prader Willi syndrome	Large fontanels Retinitis pigmentosa Hypotonia

GENERAL EXAMINATION

There are certain aspects of the general (non-neurological) examination that are of relevance to the nervous system including examination of the skin, skull, spine, and assessment for dysmorphic features and meningeal irritation signs. Skin exam is important as the skin and the nervous system have the same embryologic origin (ectoderm). Therefore, developmental CNS disorders may have associated skin signs (neurocutaneous disorders) as shown in Table **2** and Fig. **1**.

Examination of the skull for shape, fontanel size and tenseness, sutures for premature fusion (craniosynostosis) or wide separation (hydrocephalus), and sinus tenderness are important. As well, skull auscultation for bruits may indicate an underlying arteriovenous malformation. For this purpose, the bell of the stethoscope should be placed over the fontanels, eyes, and sides of the head. Examination of the spine for deformities (scoliosis, lordosis, gibbus) or midline lesions (defect, hair tuft, or lipoma) may indicate an underlying spinal dysraphism. Many syndromes may have associated CNS anomalies or features. It is important therefore to carefully assess the patient for dysmorphic features (face, mouth, palate, hands, and feet). Finally examination for meningeal irritation signs is important, including Kernig and Brudzinski signs. Neck stiffness may indicate meningitis, meningoencephalitis, subarachnoid hemorrhage, or cerebellar herniation.

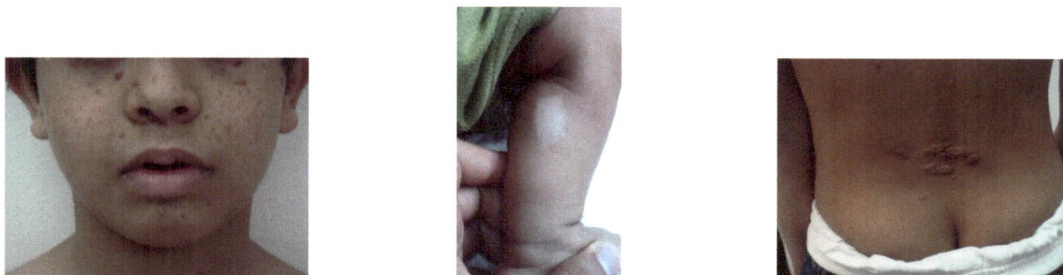

Figure 1: Adenoma sebaceum (face), ash-leaf spots (leg), and shagreen patches (lower back) are characteristic of tuberous sclerosis.

Table 2: Cutaneous features of common neurocutaneous syndromes.

Syndrome	Inheritance	Skin manifestations
Neurofibromatosis Type 1	AD	Café-au-lait spots Neurofibromas Axillary or inguinal freckling
Tuberous Sclerosis	AD	Adenoma sebaceum Ash-leaf spots Fibrous plaques Shagreen patches Periungual fibroma
Sturge Weber syndrome	Sporadic	Facial angioma (port-wine stain)
Ataxia Telangiectasia	AR	Telangiectasias (eyes, ears, cubital, and popliteal fossas)
Linear Naevus syndrome	Sporadic	Sebaceous naevus Verrucous naevus Acanthosis nigricans

In children with coma or head injury assessment of the level of consciousness is needed. The Glasgow Coma Scale quantifies the degree of responsiveness after head injury (Table **3**). A normal awake child scores 15 and a brain dead child scores 3. In head injury, scores of 8 or less correlate with severe injury.

Table 3: Glasgow coma scale (total score = 15).

Examination Section	Scores
Eye Opening	4
Spontaneously	3
To speech	2
To pain	1
None	
Best Motor Response	
Obeys	6
Localizes	5
Withdraws	4
Abnormal flexion	3
Abnormal extension	2
None	1

Table 3: cont….

Verbal Response	
Oriented	5
Confused conversation	4
Inappropriate words	3
Incomprehensible sounds	2
None	1

MENTAL STATUS EXAMINATION

Detailed assessment may be difficult in young children, however, the mini mental status examination can be done in older children and adults as shown in Table **4**. This is a screening test that includes a series of questions and commands to assess various higher cortical functions including orientation, registration, attention, calculation, recall, and language. Cognitive impairment is considered if the total score is less than 23. It is important to stress that this is only a screening test and more detailed assessments are needed if it was abnormal. The test may also miss subtle or selective cognitive impairment, particularly in executive functions.

Table 4: The mini-mental status examination (total score = 30*).

Examination Item	Score
Orientation to time, date, day, month, and year	1 point each
Orientation to place (ward, hospital, district, city, country)	1 point each
Registration (name 3 objects and ask the patient to repeat)	1 point each
Attention and calculation (subtract 7s from 100)	5 points
Recall (repeat the 3 objects named in registration)	1 point each

Language:
 	
      Name 2 objects (*e.g.* pen and watch)
      Repeat a sentence
      3 step verbal command
      1 step written command
      Write a sentence
      Draw intersecting pentagons
	1 point each
	1 point
	1 point each
	1 point
	1 point
	1 point

*Patient is considered cognitively impaired if the total score is <23.

CRANIAL NERVE ASSESSMENT

Olfactory Nerve (I)

To test smell, each nostril should be examined separately (by blocking the other nostril). The examiner should use familiar odors (*e.g.* mint, vanilla, or coffee). Avoid irritant smell, which will stimulate the fifth cranial nerve (responsible for withdrawal). Upper respiratory tract infections are the commonest cause of hyposmia (reduced smell) or anosmia (complete loss of smell). Other causes include frontal brain tumor or skull fractures involving the cribriform plate.

Optic Nerve (II)

Five modalities should be examined (visual acuity, fields, pupillary reflex, fundi, and color vision). Snellen chart should be used for visual acuity testing. The patient should read the chart from a distance of 20 feet (6 meters), alternately covering one eye, then the other. Pocket-size charts held at 14 inches from the patient's eyes can be used if wall charts are not available. If the patient wears glasses, he should be tested while he is wearing them. The test should be conducted with adequate illumination. If the patient cannot read the largest letter, finger counting and hand motion detection should be performed. Visual field testing is commonly assessed using the confrontation test, which is a crude screening method to detect major visual field defects. Another technique involves finger counting in all 4-field quadrants with one eye covered. Presenting two simultaneous visual stimuli could detect homonomous visual neglect. Direct and consensual pupillary reflex should be tested after dimming the room light. Remember that the afferent limb is 2nd and efferent is 3rd cranial nerve. Marcus gun pupil (afferent pupillary defect) results from a lesion in the optic nerve. This will result in slow pupillary dilatation (rather than quick constriction) on the affected side when the consensual reflex is tested. Finally fundal examination is important to examine the optic disc, vessels, and macula.

Occulomotor, Trochlear, and Abducent nerves (III, IV, and VI)

Inspect the eyelids for ptosis (III). Test eye movements (smooth pursuit and saccades) by asking the patient to follow an object (*e.g.* fingertip) moving in the horizontal, vertical and oblique planes. Remember that the rectus muscles move the eyes in the direction of their names (*e.g.* the medial rectus moves the eye medially). The oblique muscles move the eyes in the opposite direction (*e.g.* the superior oblique moves the eye inferiorly). As well, the superior oblique muscle moves the eye inward and the inferior oblique muscle moves the eye outward in a rotatory movement. Trochlear nerve palsy results in vertical diplopia while abducent nerve palsy results in horizontal diplopia. Test accommodation by bringing an object slowly closer to the fixating eyes looking for convergence and miosis.

Trigeminal Nerve (V)

As discussed under the sensory examination, pain and touch sensation should be examined in the V1, V2, and V3 bilaterally. Testing for the corneal reflex, particularly in patients with disturbed level of consciousness will examine two cranial nerves, afferent (V1) and efferent (VII). Teeth clenching is used to examine the masseters and temporalis muscles and lateral jaw movements for the pterygoids. Jaw reflex (5th nerve constitutes both afferent and efferent limbs) is exaggerated in patients with frontal lobe dysfunction (release reflex), or in extrapyramidal disorders (*e.g.* Parkinson's disease).

Facial Nerve (VII)

Examination of the muscles of facial expressions includes mainly the frontalis, nasalis, orbicularis oculi and oris muscles. Remember that an upper motor neuron lesion will spare the frontalis and orbicularis oculi muscles because of bilateral corticobulbar innervations while a lower motor neuron lesion (*e.g.* Bell's palsy) will involve both upper and lower halves. As well, examine taste on the anterior 2/3 of the tongue using cotton swabs soaked with salted or sweetened water applied to the tongue's lateral sides. During this test, each half should be tested separately with the tongue held out of the mouth to avoid stimulating other taste receptors in the oropharynx.

Vestibulococclear Nerve (VIII)

Assessment of balance and hearing, which may requires the use of a bell, soft voice, or a tuning fork. A simple hearing test involves rubbing the index and thumb fingers together close to each ear. Rinne and Weber tests are performed using a 512 Hz tuning fork.

Glossopharyngeal & Vagus Nerves (IX, X)

Examine the gag reflex (afferent IX and efferent X) by touching the posterior pharynx using a tongue depressor. Examine the soft palate movements (watching the uvula while saying "Ahh"). In unilateral palatal weakness, remember that the uvula will deviate towards the normal side during palatal movements.

Spinal Accessory Nerve (XI)

Shoulder drop or asymmetry may appear on the side of trapezius muscle weakness. Shrugging the shoulders will reveal ipsilateral weakness. Examine the sternocleidomastoid muscle by asking the patient to turn the head laterally against resistance. Note that the left muscle will turn the head to the right.

Hypoglossal Nerve (XII)

The tongue should be inspected for bulk and fasiculations, which may be detected only in the tongue particularly in children. This is true because of the absence of subcutaneous fat. Protruding the tongue and pushing against the examiner's finger through the cheeks will examine normal movements and power. Unilateral paralysis will result in tongue deviation towards the weak side.

Motor System

Gait assessment includes observing the patient walk normally and run. Beginning sometime between 4 to 6 years of age, most normal children will participate in a screening motor examination. Before that age, the examination should be informal and depends heavily on observation according to the child's acquired motor skills. The examiner should observe the arms for swinging and the feet for heel strike (the heel normally strikes the floor before the forefoot). Functional power assessment will include tiptoe and heel walk, hopping on one foot, and Gower's sign. Gower's sign is the inability to rise from a sitting position without holding an object for support including the patient's own body. A positive sign suggests proximal lower limb muscle weakness. Inspection of various muscle groups for (bulk, atrophy, fasiculations, chorea, tremor, myoclonus), or maintained posturing or deformity is important followed by palpation for muscle firmness, tenderness, tone, or palpable nerves. Calf muscle hypertrophy is commonly seen in duchenne muscular dystrophy. In coma, decerebrate (limb extension) posturing suggests subcortical insult, while decorticate (limb flexion) posturing suggests diffuse cortical insult. Assessment of power is also important and a specific grading system should be followed. It includes 6 categories:

1. No contraction

2. Contraction with minimal movement

3. Movement with gravity

4. Movement against gravity

5. Movement against some resistance

6. Meaning movement against full resistance (normal power)

Recognizing subtle limb weakness is fundamental to the motor examination as it may be the first sign of an upper motor neuron lesion. Apraxia is the inability to perform a given task inspite of lack of weakness. Deep tendon reflexes are critical in localizing the site of lesion as shown in Table **5**.

Table 5: Localization of some important deep tendon reflexes. A reflex is considered present (+1), normal (+2), brisk (+3), or pathological (+4).

Reflex	Muscle involved	Nerve supply	Root supply
Biceps	Biceps	Musculocutaneous	C5, C6
Triceps	Triceps	Radial	C6, C7, C8
Pectoralis	Pectoralis Major	Pectoral	C6, C7, C8
Brachioradialis	Brachioradialis	Radial	C5, C6
Finger flexors	Flexor Digitorum	Median & Ulnar	C7, C8, T1
Knee	Quadriceps Femoris	Femoral	L2, L3, L4
Adductor	Adductors	Obturator	L2, L3, L4
Ankle	Soleus/Gastrocnemius	Sciatic/Tibial	S1, S2
Planter	Small foot muscles	Plantar	L5, S1, S2

Deep tendon reflexes are important for differentiating upper *versus* lower motor neuron lesion weakness as shown in Table **6**. Exaggerated reflexes are considered pathological (+4) if associated with spasticity, clonus, or reflex spread (*e.g.* hip adduction on tapping the knee jerk or finger flexion on tapping the biceps).

It is important to note that preterm infants, particularly those less than 33 weeks of gestation, have decreased elicitation rates for patellar and biceps reflexes and have decreased overall reflex intensity when compared with their older counter parts.

Table 6: Differention of upper and lower motor neuron lesions.

Feature	UMNL	LMNL
Site of the lesion	Cerebrum hemispheres, cerebellum, brain stem, or spinal cord	Anterior horn cell, roots, nerves, neuromuscular junction, or muscles
Muscle weakness	Quadriplegia, hemiplegia, diplegia, triplegia	Proximal (myopathy) Distal (neuropathy)
Muscle tone	Spasticity/Rigidity	Hypotonia
Fasiculations	Absent	Present (tongue)
Tendon reflexes	Hyperreflexia	Hypo/areflexia
Abdominal reflexes	Absent (depending on the involved spinal level)	Present
Sensory loss	Cortical sensations	Peripheral sensations
Electromyography	Normal nerve conduction Decreased interference pattern and firing rate	Slow nerve conduction Large motor units Fasiculations and fibrillations

DEVELOPMENTAL REFLEXES

Developmental reflexes are important reflexes that can be elicited in young infants. Table 7 shows a summary of these reflexes with normal ages of appearance and disappearance. They are abnormal when absent or weak (diffuse brain insults or drug effects). However, the reflexes that appears at birth are vigorous and complete only at term and may be weak or absent in the preterm (<37 weeks gestation) infant. If these reflexes persist or become exaggerated they may indicate upper motor neuron lesion. As well, asymmetry may be abnormal. For example, asymmetric Moro reflex may indicate hemiplegia, brachial plexus injury, shoulder dislocation, or fractured humerous or clavicle.

Table 7: Important normal developmental reflexes.

Developmental reflex	Age of development	Age of disappearance
Truncal incurvation	Birth	1-2 months
Rooting	Birth	3 months
Moro	Birth	5-6 months
Tonic neck	Birth	5-6 months
Palmar grasp	Birth	6 months
Adductor spread	Birth	7-8 months
Plantar grasp	Birth	9-10 months
Landa	5-10 months	24 months
Parachute	8-9 months	Persist

CEREBELLAR EXAMINATION

Examination of coordination starts by examining the gait. In cerebellar disease, the patient is off balance with eyes open and worse with eye closure (see later under sensory examination). Walking on a straight line will identify unilateral hemispheric cerebellar disease as the patient will sway towards the affected side. Tandem walk (walking on a straight line with feet closely attached and alternating in front of each other) is more difficult to perform and may identify subtle cerebellar ataxia. Finger nose or heel shin test, rapid alternate hand movements or foot tap will test for limb ataxia. Note that the arms have to be adequately stretched during the finger nose test to identify intention tremor as the amplitude of this tremor increases as it reaches the target.

SENSORY SYSTEM

There are three main sensory modalities to be examined: 1) special sensations (discussed under cranial nerves), 2) general sensations (light touch, superficial pain, temperature, vibration and proprioception), and 3) cortical sensations (graphesthesia, stereognosis, neglect, and 2-point discrimination). Abnormalities of general sensations result from lesions in the lower motor neuron. Light touch should be tested using a napkin tip or a twisted tip of cotton wool, working from the insensitive toward the sensitive area. In the case of a hypersensitive area, the direction of testing should be reversed to minimize discomfort. One of the common pitfalls is to rapidly move the tip of the cotton in a linear or circular manner. This results in a stronger tickling sensation and detection of motion by cutaneous hair. Therefore milder degrees of sensory loss can be missed. In general both sides of the body and corresponding limbs should always be checked in an alternating fashion for comparison. Regarding pain sensation a disposable pin should be used (*e.g.* safety pin). The use of needles should be discouraged as they are designed to penetrate the skin and therefore may result in injury. The same rule of applying the stimuli from the analgesic area and working outwards should be followed. The area of sensory defect should be outlined by a series of dots with the patient's eyes closed. Use irregular stimulus timing so the patient does not know when to expect the next touch or pinprick. If the sensory defect is hysterical, inconsistencies in the marking will be revealed easily. Other sensations include temperature, which can be checked using test tubes full of warm and cold water. In practice, the metal part of the patellar hammer or stethoscope is usually cold and can be used for as a screening test. For vibration sense a 128 Hz tuning fork should be applied over the distal bony prominences followed by more proximal testing with eyes closed. The examiner should teach the patient what to expect before performing the test as some may report the pressure rather than vibration sensation. Romberg sign will help in testing position sense as the patient stands with outstretched hands and closely placed feet. Off balance with eye closure represents a positive sign, indicating sensory ataxia. Regarding abnormal cortical sensations, they result from an upper motor neuron lesion usually involving the right parietal lobe. Abnormal cortical sensations include agraphesthesia (inability to identify written numbers or letters on the patient's skin, *e.g.* palms), astereognosis (inability to identify an object placed in the patient's hand, *e.g.* key), neglect (inability to identify one of two simultaneous stimulation points), and 2 point discrimination (particularly on the finger tips), all performed with eye closure.

SUMMARY

This chapter presented a concise and simple outline for the examination of the nervous system. Different techniques of eliciting physical signs and possible pitfalls in the examination were discussed. Although many students and residents will continue to consider examining the nervous system as one of the most difficult parts of the physical examination, we hope that in this review certain problems like organizing a complete examination, and eliciting and interpreting neurological signs were highlighted and clarified. Repeated examinations, preferably in conjunction with another colleague for instructive criticism, will remain the key for successfully and consistently eliciting the various neurological signs.

BIBLIOGRAPHY

Jan MMS, Al-Buhairi AR, Baeesa SS: Concise Outline of the Nervous System Examination for the Generalist. Neurosciences 2001;6(1):16-22.

Jan MMS: Neurological Examination of Difficult and Poorly Cooperative Children. J Child Neurol 2007;22(10):1209-13.

Jan MMS, Khalifa MA. Nervous System and Development. In: Alhowasi MN (ed). Manual of Clinical Pediatrics. 4th Edition, Medical Book House, Riyadh, Saudi Arabia, p130-176, 2007.

Jan MM: Facial Paralysis: A Presenting Feature of Rhabdomyosarcoma. Int J Pediatr Otorhinolaryngol 1998;46:221-224.

Jan MM: An Unusual Cause of Isolated Trochlear Nerve Palsy. Neurosciences 2007;12(2):149-151.

CHAPTER 3

Examining the Difficult Child

Abstract: Children are generally more difficult to examine when compared to adults. As well, physicians are usually judged by parents according to their skills in examining their children. Difficult and poorly cooperative children remain the most challenging group to examine accurately and completely. The physician becomes less confident and the neurological signs questionable if the child was uncooperative. Certainly, repeated examinations and experience play an important role; however, solid knowledge, strong communication skills, accurate observation skills, and use of proper techniques are crucial for eliciting and interpreting neurological signs in difficult children. In this chapter, I present some practical tips and skills that can be utilized to improve the likelihood of obtaining accurate information about the neurological status of young and difficult children.

Keywords: Neurological, Examination, General, Difficult, Cerebellum, Uncooperative, Signs, Organization, Cranial nerves, Motor, Sensory.

THE DIFFICULT CHILD

Many children view physicians as threatening and feel hostility towards hospitals. Parents can contribute to the stress of their children when visiting a physician. Fear and anxiety from doctors and needles can be easily reflected to the child. Our Saudi culture may have an additional negative influence as the doctor's visit is frequently used as a punishment threat and correlated with pain and needles. Several factors were found predictive of difficult behavior during the evaluation including problems on visiting a previous physician, anxiety when meeting unfamiliar people, not enough time to adjust to the medical situation, fear of injections, and parental fear of physicians. In another study, negative behaviors were associated with younger child's age, learning or behavioral problems, and history of hospitalization. It appears that both child's temperament and conditioning factors play important role in the development of their fear from physicians. The developmental stage is also important as children between 2-5 years are more likely to be uncooperative and therefore difficult to examine. Stranger's anxiety usually develops after 6 months of age and becomes stronger with advancing age. Therefore, the very young infant and older child are relatively easier to examine. The young uncooperative child may not necessarily be afraid, but rather hungry, dirty, or in pain. Understanding these factors and patience are important in order to conduct a detailed and accurate examination. Additional contributing factors to resistance and defiance include the underlying neurological condition resulting in irritability, confusion or behavioral disorder. Children with developmental or cognitive deficits are also at higher risk of being poorly cooperative. A patient and empathetic physician and a supportive guiding parent are needed to prevent excessive fear.

TIPS DURING HISTORY TAKING

Proper interaction and good communication with the parents is critical as parental behavior has often been cited as a crucial factor in children's ability to cope in stressful situations. The physician should use the time during history taking to inspect the child for any clues of neurological impairment (Table **1**). Many organs and functions can be assessed reasonably well by inspection, observation, and behavioral responses. Keep the child next to the parent during the interview and avoid approaching him or her in the beginning of the evaluation. It would be advisable to avoid wearing the white lab coat and dress in a familiar way. It is also useful to present a small toy or a treat in the beginning of the visit after getting the parents permission. Preparatory play with parental involvement before and at the beginning of the examination could improves their coping and ease the child's stress. Smile, behave in a friendly manner, and maintain intermittent eye contact with the child to decrease her or his anxiety and improve the cooperation. The child should then realize that the physician does not represent a direct threat.

Table 1: Summary of the tips for examining the difficult child.

During History Taking	1- Keep the child next to the parent
	2- Observe the child carefully
	3- Smile, be friendly, and maintain eye contact
	4- Avoid wearing the white lab coat
	5- Start interacting with the child
Beginning of Interaction	1- Present a small toy or a treat
	2- Hands off, use observation
	3- Keep the younger child in the mothers lap
	4- Let the parents do the undressing
	5- Do not show your tools
During the Examination	1- Start with the most relevant system
	2- Be focused
	3- Use your observation skills starting with gait
	4- Make the parents as an example for testing
	5- Leave invasive or painful tests to the end
During Procedures	1- Invite parents to attend
	2- Prepare child and parent for their role
	3- Use the treatment room with pain control
	4- Position the child in a comfortable manner
	5- Maintain a calm and positive atmosphere

TIPS DURING THE EXAMINATION

Evidence suggests that patient anxiety and poor cooperation are socio-psychological in origin. Ongoing communication and adequate information to both parents and child during examination procedures can reduce their anxiety; uncooperative behavior, examination time, and misunderstanding that cause a poor professional image. Detailed and long examination may be difficult to perform in an uncooperative child. Only focused examination may be possible, concentrating on the most relevant aspects (*e.g.* motor system in a child with cerebral palsy). Clues from the history should guide the focused examination. Many neurological signs can be identified by careful observation. For example, the child may not cooperate for detailed cranial nerve examination, however, a squint, drooling, or facial asymmetry may be evident, particularly in a crying child. Inspection of the tongue and palatal movements is easily done in a screaming child. Combativeness may be a good sign of normal power and escaping or climbing on the mother indicate coordination and motor abilities. In a less difficult child, certain tips are helpful in improving the cooperation (Table **1**). Do not show your tools that may be viewed as a threat by the scared child. The physician may use the parents as an example to show that tendon reflexes will not hurt and may give such tools to the child to look at and feel assured that they are not harmful. You may also ask the parent to perform certain tasks such as undressing or removing the shoes. Interact and play with the child as you try to examine him or her. Leave uncomfortable components, such as planter's response, to the end. We frequently ask the parents to take the child for a walk in the clinic or the corridor for gait and power assessment.

ORGANIZATION OF CORE EXAMINATION

An organized approach, as outlined in chapter 2, may not be possible in an uncooperative child. Performing a focused examination is better than a skipped incomplete examination in the difficult child. Proceed to the system related to the main complaint (*e.g.* motor system in cerebral palsy) before examining less relevant aspects of the examination. An experienced clinician knows exactly what to look for at the beginning of the examination and is usually confident about what to expect to find. Mental status can be assessed based on the history and level of alertness and interaction. Behavioral abnormalities such as inattention or hyperactivity can be observed. Most cranial nerves can be examined by observation alone, *e.g.* eye movements, fixation, facial, tongue and palatal movements. As well, motor system can be examined by careful examination of the gait. Power can be assessed by giving a toy and then try to take it back to check resistance. A small toy can also be used to assess coordination and cerebellar testing. Sensory examination should be left to the end. Note that this examination is difficult even in the cooperative child. Leave pain testing to the end and always examine for consistency. A complete examination of the difficult and poorly cooperative child will take more time. Students and less experienced physicians usually spend a greater proportion of time in examining their patients than senior physicians and consultants. This may not be practical in busy practice or during clinical examinations where time is limited. The performance of medical students and their time management will improve if neurological examination is observed by a trained neurologist, who is then able to provide immediate feedback to the student. Junior physicians certainly will handle difficult children better with more experience. My advice is not to spend too much time after examining the most relevant aspects as a higher incidence of correct diagnosis and more effective management does not necessarily follow if the doctor is allowed more time. Physicians have been shown to generate the correct hypothesis early, usually within the first five minutes of the clinical interview. Many children could have had the correct diagnosis made only on the basis of their history. As well, the length of time spent with the patient was not as critical as effective communication in a walk-in pediatric clinic. Many children with common neurological disorders, such as migraine and epilepsy, may have normal physical examination. However, more time has to be spent in difficult and complicated disorders in order to make a comprehensive assessment.

COOPERATION DURING PROCEDURES

Medical procedures can be unpleasant experiences for children and their parents. Many of difficult and uncooperative children became so after a difficulty with an invasive procedure such as those that involve pain or needles. In special situations where children need repeated examinations or procedures, coping-skills training could reduce their anxiety. A clinical psychologist trained in behavioral psychology, communication, motivation and control techniques, would help in the inpatient or outpatient setting. Several strategies can be used to help increase the comfort of infants and children and also the parents and medical staff during invasive procedures as shown in Table **1**. They include; 1) preparing the child and parent for the procedure and for their role during the procedure, 2) inviting the parent or caregiver to be present, 3) utilizing the treatment room for stressful procedures, 4) positioning the child in a comfortable manner, and 5) maintaining a calm and positive atmosphere. Careful attention is needed for pain control to make the experience even less traumatic and prevent future negative behaviors, however, most difficulties arise when the parents and child do not know what to expect or do during such procedures. This remains a problem, particularly in our region. Our recent Saudi Study revealed that adequate explanations for the ordered investigations and treatments were received by only 78% and 69% of parents respectively. The authors concluded that physicians need to pay more attention towards providing explanations and guidance for the ordered investigations and treatments.

SUMMARY

Many physicians consider examining the nervous system one of the most difficult parts of the physical examination. Difficult and poorly cooperative children remain the most challenging group to examine accurately and completely. In this chapter, I presented some practical tips and techniques that can be utilized to improve the likelihood of obtaining accurate information about the neurological status of young and difficult children. A patient and empathetic physician and a supportive guiding parent are needed to prevent excessive fear.

BIBLIOGRAPHY

Jan MMS: Neurological Examination of Difficult and Poorly Cooperative Children. J Child Neurol 2007;22(10):1209-13.

CHAPTER 4

Normal Development

Abstract: In this chapter various aspects of normal development and assessment will be discussed. Development is a continuous process by which one acquires learned skills. Ongoing development results from the myelination process, as well as, synaptogenesis and organization of the nervous system. Developmental history is divided into gross motor, fine motor, language (receptive and expressive), and psychosocial skills. Wide variations exist in the development of normal milestones. For example, males tend to be faster in acquiring motor skills while females are faster in acquiring verbal skills.

Keywords: Neurological, Examination, General, Development, Assessment, Evaluation, Gross, Fine, Language, Social, Adaptive.

DEVELOPMENTAL ASSESSMENT

Objective assessment of cognitive functions including IQ can be performed with accuracy only after 3-5 years of age. Before that age, we mainly rely on developmental milestones. Development follows an orderly progress, usually in a cephalo-caudal direction (head control, sitting, then standing). In other words, a child cannot sit if there is no head control or rolling. No child can walk before attaining the sitting position. Development of a particular skill requires loss of certain primitive reflexes. Persistence of tonic neck reflex can interfere with normal sitting. For the premature infant, the assessed developmental level should be adjusted in relation to chronological age during the first years of life. During developmental examination one should be observant and try to collect as much information as possible without disturbing the child. If the child is able to perform a specific skill, proceed to test for the next skill (*e.g.* if the child is walking, test for running and hoping). Important developmental milestones should be remembered. There is a wide range of age for the achievement of various developmental milestones (Table **1**). Wider variation is expected for language skills. Delay is considered only if the upper age range is exceeded without attaining a given milestone. Mild abnormal variations should be taken with respect to family history. Certain families are known to have a normally earlier or later age of milestones (*e.g.* early or late talkers, early or late walkers). It may not be always possible to assess the developmental age by one examination, especially when the child is uncooperative. Further assessment on follow-up visits would be needed in this situation.

Tables 1 (A-G): Important normal developmental milestones:

A- 6 weeks – 3 months

Gross motor	Head control (2-3 months)
	Ventral suspension (head held in the level of the body briefly at 2 months and lifted up by 3 months)
Fine motor and vision	Fixate at mother's or examiner's face
	Follows horizontally to 90°
Language	Respond to rattle or bell held at the ear level by turning to the sound
	Startle response
Social behavior	Smiles (6 weeks)
	Turns to regard the observer's face

B- 4-8 months

Gross motor	Bears weight on legs while held upright
	Downward parachute response (4 - 6 months)
	Can be pulled to sit (5 months)
	Sits with support (6 months)
	Sits without support (7 months)
	Forward parachute response (7 months)
	Crawls (8 months)

Table 1: cont…..

Fine motor and vision	Reaches out to grasp (palmar grasp, 4-5 months) Transfers objects from hand to hand (6 months) Fixes on small objects Follows falling toys
Language	Vocalizes (5 months) Polysyllabic babbling (7 months) Responds to whisper at ear level
Social behavior	Puts everything to mouth Hand and foot regard Strangers anxiety (6 months) Plays peek-a-boo

C- 8-12 months

Gross motor	Pulls to standing position) Walks holding furniture Walks alone (10-14 months)
Fine motor and vision	Points with index finger Casts (throws) Pincer grasp (11-13 months) Holds 2 bricks and bangs them together
Language	Turns to sound Uses "mama" and "dada" Understands several words
Social behavior	Drinks from cup Indicates needs Plays pat-a-cake Waves bye-bye

D- 1–2 years

Gross motor	Walks backwards Carries toys while walking Climbs onto chair Climbs stairs with 2 feet per step holding the rail
Fine motor and vision	Pincer grasp (11-13 months) Scribbles Turns pages Builds tower of 3 or 4 bricks
Language	Jabbers continually Utters 3 or more words other than mama and dada Points to eyes, nose and mouth Obeys simple instructions (1 step command)
Social behavior	Holds spoon: gets food to mouth Explores environment Takes off shoes and socks Indicates toilet needs

E- 2–3 years

Gross motor	Climbs stairs unaided with one foot per step and descends with 2 feet per step Jumps in place Kicks a ball (2 years)

Table 1: cont…..

Fine motor and vision	Understand hundreds and thousands Copies a vertical line Hand preference (2 years) Builds tower of 8 bricks
Language	Uses plurals Gives name
Social behavior	Plays alone Eats with spoon and fork Puts on clothes Dry throughout day

F- 3–4 years

Gross motor	Runs fast Climbs stairs in adult manner Paddles tricycle (3 years) Stands on one foot (3 years)
Fine motor and vision	Copies a circle Threads beads well Matches 2 colors
Language	Uses prepositions Uses sentences of 4 words Gives full name, sex and age
Social behavior	Eats with knife and fork Goes to toilet alone Dresses with supervision Washes and dries hands Separates from mother easily Stool continence

G- 4-5 years

Gross motor	Hops on one foot well Climbs ladder, tree, slide Walks heel-to-toe Bounces and catches ball
Fine motor and vision	Copies cross and square Copies a triangle Draws a man with main feature Build a bridge of 3 bricks Draw man with 3 parts
Language	Speaks grammatically Counts up to 10 Recognizes colors
Social behavior	Shares toys Comforts a friend in distress Brushes teeth Dresses without supervision Dry day and night

DEVELOPMENTAL REFLEXES

Developmental reflexes are important normal reflexes that can be elicited in young infants as summarized in Table **7** in Chapter **2**. Developmental reflexes can be abnormal when absent or weak (diffuse brain insults or drug effects). However, the reflexes that appears at birth are vigorous and complete only at term and may be weak or absent in the preterm (<37 weeks gestation) infant. If these reflexes persist or become exaggerated they may indicate upper motor neuron lesion. As well, asymmetry may be abnormal. For example, asymmetric Moro reflex may indicate hemiplegia, brachial plexus injury, shoulder dislocation, or fractured humerus or clavicle.

BIBLIOGRAPHY

Jan MMS, Al-Buhairi AR, Baeesa SS: Concise Outline of the Nervous System Examination for the Generalist. Neurosciences 2001;6(1):16-22.

CHAPTER 5

Developmental Disorders

Abstract: Developmental disorders are a group of early and chronic disorders affecting 5-10% of children. Developmental delay is a subtype defined as significant delay in two or more of the following developmental domains: motor (gross and fine), language (receptive an expressive), cognition, social and adaptive activities. The estimated prevalence of global developmental delay is 1-3% of children younger than 5 years. Developmental delay is a clinical presentation of a wide variety of congenital or acquired etiologies. It results in significant learning deficits incompatable with the child's chronological age. Significant delay in a given developmental domain is defined as performance two standard deviations or more below the mean for age. The term developmental delay is usually reserved for younger children (less than 5 years of age), whereas the term mental retardation is usually applied to older children when IQ testing is more reliable.

Keywords: Neurological, Development, Disorders, Assessment, Delay, Regression, Evaluation, Mental retardation, Genetic, Metabolic.

INTRODUCTION

A child with developmental delay is not always destined to be mentally retarded. Infants and children may have delayed developmental that may have predominant motor deficits, such as cerebral palsy or neuromuscular disorders, with minimal or no cognitive deficits. The diagnosis of mental retardation (see later in the chapter) requires accurate assessment of intelligence, which is not possible in infants and young children. Available instruments for assessing intelligence (such as the Stanford-Binet or Wechsler Preschool Primary Scale of Intelligence) are not suitable for children younger than 3 years of age.

ETIOLOGY

In up to 70% of patients, the etiology for developmental delay remains unknown. However, accurate identification of the underlying causes has important implications for predicting the clinical course, providing councelling, treatment, and more accurate prognostic information. The etiologic yield of various investigations is usually around 30-40%. Hoever, some reports found higher diagnostic yield depending on the extent of diagnostic work particularly using advanced genetic and neuroimaging techniques. Comprehensive history and physical examination may reveal the etiology without the need for such expensive work up. The following are important etiologies that are addressed in more detail and based on the practice parameters of the American Academy of Neurology and the Child Neurology Society recommendations published in the journal "Neurology" in 2003. Important etiologies include:

1. Unknown (commonest)

2. Perinatal insult (trauma, hypoxia, infection)

3. Genetic disorders (chromosomal, syndromic)

4. Hypothyroidism

5. Metabolic disorders

Genetic Disorders

Genetic disorders are usually suspected during the physical examination (Fig **1**). The overall yield of cytogenetic testing (karyotyping) in children with global developmental delay is around 4%. Some of the common diagnoses include Down syndrome, sex chromosome aneuploidies (47, XXY), fragile X syndrome, and unbalanced translocations/deletion syndromes. The diagnostic yield may reach 20% if the child has dysmorphic features or other congenital anomalies. Below we will discuss three important genetic etiologies including; Fragile X syndrome, Rett syndrome, and Subtelomeric chromosomal rearrangements.

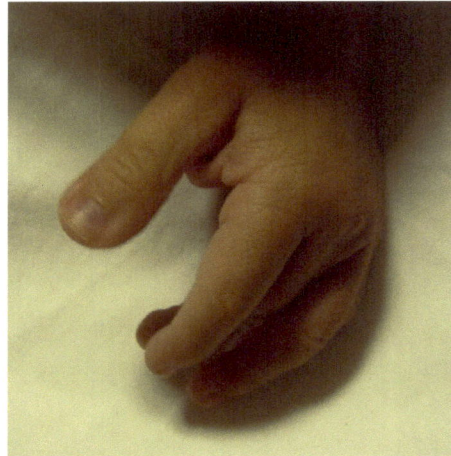

Figure 1: Big thumb in a child with Rubinstein Taybi syndrome.

Fragile X syndrome is the most common inherited disorder causing global developmental delay. It is caused by a mutation in the FMR1 gene. The diagnosis should be suspected if there is family history of mental retardation or characteristic facial features that includes long jaw, high forehead, large protuberant ears, hyperextensible joints, soft and velvety palmar skin with redundancy on the dorsum of the hand, and enlargement of the testes (macroorchidism). Children with Fragile X syndrome may have no dysmorphic features. They have shy personality with lack of eye contact followed by friendliness and verbosity. Note that regular chromosomal analysis will not diagnose this disorder. Specific molecular testing for the FMR1 mutation is diagnostic.

Rett syndrome is one of the leading causes of global developmental delay and mental retardation in females. It is caused by mutations in the X-linked gene encoding methyl-CpG-binding protein 2 (MECP2). Patients appear to develop normally until 6-18 months of age followed by gradually loss of speech and purposeful hand use, and microcephaly (Table **1**). Seizures, autistic behavior, ataxia, episodic hyperventilation, and stereotypic hand movements are characteristc. Recent studies have shown that males can also be affected.

Table 1: Diagnostic criteria for Rett syndrome.

Necessary Criteria
1- Apparently normal prenatal and perinatal period
2- Apparently normal psychomotor development in the first 6 months
3- Normal head circumference at birth
4- Deceleration of head growth between ages 5 months and 4 years
5- Loss of acquired purposeful hand skills between 6-30 months
6- Severe expressive and receptive language and psychomotor retardation
7- Stereotypic hand movements (wringing/squeezing/clapping/tapping)
8- Gait apraxia and truncal apraxia/ataxia between ages 1 and 4 years
9- Diagnosis tentative until 2 to 5 years of age
Supportive Criteria
1- Breathing dysfunction
2- EEG abnormalities
3- Seizures
4- Spasticity often associated with muscle wasting and dystonia

Table 1: cont….

5- Peripheral vasomotor disturbances
6- Scoliosis
7- Growth retardation
8- Hypotrophic small feet
Exclusion Criteria
1- Evidence of intrauterine growth retardation
2- Organomegaly or other signs of storage disease
3- Retinopathy or optic atrophy
4- Microcephaly at birth
5- Evidence of perinatally acquired brain lesion
6- Existence of identifiable metabolic or progressive disorder
7- Acquired neurological disorders from infections or head trauma

Subtelomeric chromosomal rearrangements result in small rearrangements involving the ends of chromosomes and may be associated with developmental delay. They are identified by molecular tests that include fluorescence *in situ* hybridization (FISH), subtelomeric probes, and microsatellite markers. Uniparental disomy (inheritance of both copies of one chromosome from the same parent) can be detected using this technique. However, these tests are expensive and should be used after obtaining a normal chromosomal study. Their diagnostic yield is increased with positive family history of developmental delay, prenatal onset of growth retardation, facial dysmorphic features, postnatal growth abnormalities, or other congenital abnormalities.

Causes identified by Neuroimaging

Brain MRI is more sensitive than CT in detecting developmental brain abnormalities, such as migrational disorders (Fig. **2**). Up to 50% of children with developmental delay have some MRI abnormality that explains their problems. The yield is even higher if the child has other abnormalities on examination such as microcephaly or motor deficits. In cerebral palsy, MRI is sensitive for assessing the degree of white matter abnormality which correlates with the degree of cognitive disability. Therefore, neuroimaging (pereferably MRI) is recommended routinely as part of the diagnostic evaluation of children with developmental delay.

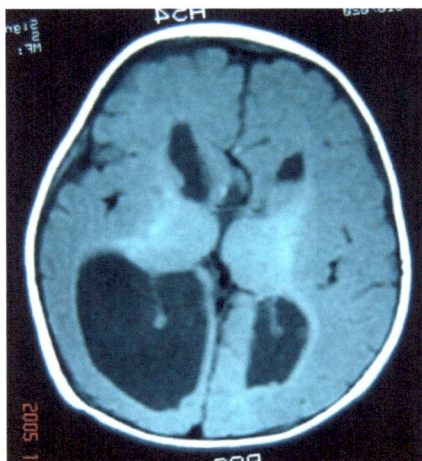

Figure 2: MRI of a girl with severe delay, infantile spasms and retinal lacunae (Aicardi syndrome) showing absent corpus callosum.

Hypothyroidism

Unrecognized or subclinical hypothyroidism is a potentially treatable cause of developmental delay. Diagnostic delay has been linked to significant long term neuro-developmental sequelae. Implementation of newborn screening programs has resulted in early recognition and therefore early treatment preventing such sequelae. Suggestive symptoms include enlarged fontanels, protruding tongue, and constipation. However, thyroid function testing (Free T4 and TSH) is usually recommended routinely in children with developmental delay or central hypotonia inorder not to miss such treatable disease.

Vision and Hearing Abnormalities

Children with developmental delay are at increased risk to have vision and hearing impairments affecting around 20% of these children. They may interfere with the developmental progress or rehabilitation effects and therefore correcting them will improve the ultimate developmental outcome. Therefore, vision and hearing assessment are indicated routinely in children with developmental delay. Ophthalmologic assessment includes visual acuity, extraocular movements, and funduscopy. Audiometric assessment may include behavioral audiometry or brainstem auditory evoked response testing. Alternatively, transient evoked otoacoustic emissions can be used when audiometry is not bpossible.

METABOLIC DISORDERS

Metabolic disorders (amino and organic acids) are usually associated with acute decompensation or regression of developmental milestones rather than developmental delay. Occasionally, early onset or severe metabolic deficits can present with developmental arrest that may be confused with static brain insults. The advent of tandem mass spectrometry for universal newborn screening programs has further reduced the yield of routine metabolic testing in infants with developmental delay. In addition to progressive course, most children with inborn errors of metabolism have other suggestive features such as hepatosplenomegaly, coarse facial features, consanguinity, similar family history, or history of unexplained neonatal death. Therefore, routine metabolic screening in children with developmental delay is not indicated.

SCREENING

Developmental surveillance is an important component of pediatric care. Routine monitoring of a child's developmental progress is recommended routinely. Children at risk (*e.g.* prematurity, psycho-social factors) for developmental delay should be targeted through these follow-up programs that can be incorporate during routine periodic assessments or vaccination visits. There is clear evidence demonstrating the benefits of such early identification on various intervention programs and ultimate developmental outcomes.

Mental Retardation

Mental retardation (MR) is impairment of cognitive functions with multiple etiologies and a broad spectrum of functional impairment and disability. It is an important public health issue because of its prevalence and the need for extensive support services. Its management requires early diagnosis and intervention, coupled with access to health care and educational resources. By definition, MR begins in childhood and is characterized by limitations in intelligence and adaptive skills. The Diagnostic and Statistical Manual IV defines MR by three co-existing criteria (significant sub-average intellectual functioning, adaptive functioning deficit, and onset before 18 years of age). The severity of cognitive impairment is characterized by the extent of deviation of the IQ below 100, the estimated mean for the population. The lower limit of normal is considered to be two standard deviations below the mean or an IQ of 70. Gradations of severity include IQs in the following ranges:

- Mild (55-70)

- Moderate (40 -55)

- Severe (25-40)

· Profound (<25)

Adaptive skills are the skills of daily living that are needed to live, work, and play in the community. They include communication, social and interpersonal skills, self-care, home living, use of community resources, self-direction, functional academic skills (reading, writing and basic mathematics), work, leisure, and health and safety. Adaptive functioning is considered to be impaired when there is a deficit in at least two of these areas compared to children of the same age and culture. The term MR usually is applied to children older than five years of age, when IQ testing is more reliable. The preferred term in younger children with significant deficits in learning skills and adaptation is global developmental delay. Global developmental delay has been defined by a practice parameter of the Quality Standards Subcommittee of the American Academy of Neurology and the Practice Committee of the Child Neurology Society as performance at least two standard deviations below the mean, using standardized norm-referenced age appropriate criteria, in at least two of the following developmental subscales: motor (gross/fine), speech and language, cognition, personal-social, and daily living skills. The terms global developmental delay and MR are not interchangeable. A child with global developmental delay will not necessarily test in the mentally retarded range when older. The incidence of MR varies among studies due to differences in study design, diagnostic approach, severity of the condition, and population characteristics. The prevalence of MR in the general population is estimated to be approximately 1%. MR is mild in approximately 85% of affected individuals. When the diagnosis is based upon IQ alone, the estimated prevalence increases to approximately 3%. However, prevalence varies with age and gender and is highest in school age and male populations. The causes of MR are extensive and include any disorder that interferes with brain development. Identifying a cause enables appropriate counseling, focused interventions, treatments, surveillance, and anticipation of possible medical or behavior complications, and the provision of a more accurate prognosis. Genetic causes have implications for family planning. Causes usually are classified according to the time of the insult, as prenatal, natal, and postnatal. When the etiology is known, prenatal causes account for most cases of MR, regardless of severity. However, the distribution of causes varies with severity. In up to 32% no etiology can be identified despite extensive evaluation. Among the known prenatal causes of MR, the majority are cytogenetic abnormalities including Fragile X syndrome, Rett syndrome, Down syndrome, and Submicroscopic subtelomeric rearrangements involving the ends of chromosomes. Important prenatal cause includes brain malformations. Less common prenatal causes include placental insufficiency (intrauterine growth retardation), congenital infection, and environmental toxins or teratogens (*e.g.* alcohol, lead, mercury, hydantoin, and valproate). Radiation exposure and unrecognized congenital hypothyroidism are associated with MR. In developing countries without newborn thyroid screening programs; congenital hypothyroidism is diagnosed in up to 3% of children with cognitive delay. Postnatal causes include complications of prematurity, hypoxic ischemic encephalopathy, infection, trauma, and intracranial hemorrhage. Some of these causes may have prenatal origins. Children with MR usually are brought to the attention of the physician because of parental concerns of language delay, immature behavior, or immature self-help skills. Parents may first recognize delayed development when a younger sibling overtakes an older child in these skills. A specific parental complaint of possible MR is unusual. Increasing severity of MR is associated with earlier presentation. Some children with mild MR may be undetected until school age. Those who have a known genetic disorder can be diagnosed in infancy, regardless of their IQ. Language development is considered a reasonably good indicator of future intelligence in a child without hearing impairment. Thus, language delay associated with global developmental delay suggests cognitive impairment. This should be distinguished from isolated familial expressive language delay, which has a more favorable prognosis. In contrast, gross motor skills are less significantly associated with cognitive delay. As the severity of MR increases, other conditions are more likely to be associated including epilepsy, motor deficits, vision and hearing impairments. In some cases, these other morbidities are the presenting features. Autistic spectrum disorder may result in MR and communication and behavioral disorder. Children with MR may appear to have attention deficit hyperactivity disorder (ADHD). ADHD usually occur in cognitively normal children, however, because of inattention, their IQ scores may be lower than expected. Children with hyperactivity or inattention resulting from MR are less likely to benefit from stimulant medications, which are indicated for ADHD. Other associations with MR include eating disorders (pica and rumination), depression, and anxiety. Depression may be manifested as aggressive or irritable externalizing behaviors. Aggressive and self-injurious behaviors are common and can result from side effects of sedative-hypnotic and neuroleptic medications. The diagnosis of MR requires an assessment of intellectual function and adaptive function. Intelligence is measured by the administration of standardized tests to compare measured performance to that expected for age. The following tests are the most commonly used including Wechsler Preschool and Primary Scale of Intelligence (WPPSI) for ages 3-7 years, Wechsler Intelligence Scales for Children (WISC III) for ages 6-12 years, and Stanford-Binet Intelligence Scale for 2-23 years. Tests used to evaluate infants include the Bayley Scales of Infant Development and the Griffiths Mental Development Scales. However, these are not considered accurate in predicting future intelligence. In general, an IQ score of 70 (two standard deviations below the mean) is considered below normal intelligence. Children too impaired or uncooperative for assessment with standard testing methods are assumed to have below average intellectual function. Children with hyperactivity, attention disorder, and language disorders may score below their potential and the results should therefore be taken with caution. Another limitation is that a child's test results may change over time. As a result, while they provide information about abilities measured at the time of the test, they are not necessarily an accurate measurement of the child's potential. IQ determination alone is an imprecise measure of a child's intellectual abilities.

BIBLIOGRAPHY

Shevell M, Ashwal S, Donley D, Flint J, Gingold M, Hirtz D, Majnemer A, Noetzel M, Sheth RD. Practice parameter: Evaluation of the child with global developmental delay. Report of the Quality Standards Subcommittee of the American Academy of Neurology and the Practice Committee of the Child Neurology Society. Neurology 2003;60(3):367-380.

Jan MMS. Pediatric Neuro-developmental and behavioral disorders: Practitioner's Perspectives. Neurosciences 2005;10(2):149-154.

Jan MM: Outcome of Bilateral Periventricular Nodular Heterotopia in Monozygotic Twins with Megalencephaly. Dev Med Child Neurol 1999;41:486-488.

Jan MM, Dooley JM, Gordon K: Male Rett Syndrome Variant: Application of The Diagnostic Criteria. Ped Neurol 1999;20(3):238-240.

Jan MM. MCQs: Aicardi syndrome. Neurosciences 2007;12(4):354-5.

CHAPTER 6

Cerebral Palsy

Abstract: Cerebral palsy (CP) is a motor disorder resulting from a non-progressive (static) insult to the developing brain. In fact, CP is a clinical presentation of a wide variety of cerebral cortical or sub-cortical insults occurring during the first year of life. Preterm infants are at the highest risk for developing CP. The vulnerable brain is harmed during a critical period of development primarily by known CNS complications of prematurity such as intraventricular hemorrhage (IVH) and periventicular leukomalacia (PVL). Children with CP suffer from multiple problems and potential disabilities that require the provision of family centered services that make a difference in the lives of these children and their families. The aim of this chapter is to provide an updated overview of CP and review the most recent advances on clinical and therapeutic interventions.

Keywords: Cerebral, Palsy, Motor, Development, Assessment, Delay Evaluation, Gross, Fine, Language, Social, Adaptive, Weakness.

EPIDEMIOLOGY

The worldwide incidence of CP is approximately 2-2.5/1000 live births. The incidence is strongly associated with gestational age occurring in 1 of 20 surviving preterm infants. It is important to note that although prematurity is the commonest risk factor for developing CP; the majority of affected children are full-term. This can be explained by the fact that there are many more full-term than preterm infants born at a given time. Despite the reduction in the rate of birth asphyxia from 40/100, 000 in 1979 to 11/100, 000 in 1996, no associated reduction in the prevalence or incidence of CP was seen. In fact, the prevalence of CP in the USA has increased by 20% (from 1.9 to 2.3/1000 live births) between 1960 and 1986. This increase is likely related to the survival of very low birth weight premature infants. There is also evidence of associated increase in the severity of disability. This emphasizes the need for more efforts to decrease rate of prematurity in addition to decreasing the associated neurological injury among these infants.

CLINICAL MANIFESTATIONS AND CLASSIFICATION

Children with CP usually present with developmental delay and motor deficits. The distinction between static (non-progressive) and progressive clinical course is very important. Classically, loss of previously acquired milestones (regression) marks the onset of most metabolic and neurodegenerative disorders (NDD). However, some NDD or metabolic disorders have a slow rate of progression and can be misdiagnosed as CP. Therefore, clear developmental regression may not be evident, particularly in the early stages of the disease or at a younger age of onset. As well, the neurological consequences of CP may be delayed for several months because of the immaturity of the nervous system. Motor deficits of CP include negative phenomena such as weakness, fatigue, incoordination and positive phenomena such as spasticity, clonus, rigidity, and spasms. Spasticity is a velocity dependent increased muscle tone with hyperreflexia resulting from hyperexcitability of the stretch reflex. It can lead to muscle stiffness and functional impairment. If not treated, it can progress to muscle fibrosis, contractures, and subsequent musculoskeletal deformities. CP can be classified according to the severity of motor deficits as mild, moderate, or severe. Several other classification systems exist based on pathophysiology, etiology, and distribution of motor deficits as follow.

1- Pathophysiologic classification

Insults resulting in neuronal loss can be 1) cortical (pyramidal) resulting in spasticity, 2) basal ganglial (extrapyramidal) resulting in abnormal movements such as choreoathetosis, 3) cerebellar resulting in hypotonia, or 4) mixed. Spastic CP is the most common type accounting for up to 75% of cases. A smaller percentage of children with CP demonstrate extrapyramidal (dyskinetic) features, including combinations of athetosis, chorea, and dystonia. The abnormal movements usually develop in the second year of life and become most apparent during volitional motor activities with associated speech impairments. Most children with extrapyramidal CP have normal intelligence; however, their abilities can be underestimated due to the severity of their motor and communication deficits. Kernicterus (bilirubin encephalopathy) is a leading cause of extrapyramidal CP. The affected neonate appears weak, listless, and hypotonic, with poor feeding. Over a period of months, hypertonia, opisthotonos, chroeoathetosis, and sensorineural hearing loss develops. Hypotonic cerebral palsy occurs rarely; however, most children progress to other CP subtypes. Mixed CP occurs when the child displays a combination of features, such as spasticity and choreoathetosis.

2- Etiologic Classification

Up to 50% of CP cases have no identifiable underlying etiology. The etiologies can be classified according the timing of the insult as prenatal (commonest), natal, or postnatal. Another etiologic classification system depends on the actual cause such as congenital (developmental, malformations, syndromic) or acquired (traumatic, infectious, hypoxic, ischemic, TORCH infections etc). Perinatal asphyxia is a cause in only 8-15% of all cases. Most of these children have clinical features of neonatal hypoxic ischemic encephalopathy HIE such as disturbed level of consciousness, seizures, and other end organ dysfunction. Although a normal cord pH excludes HIE, a pH of <7.0 is associated with encephalopathy in only 15% of infants. Similarly, apgar scores are predictive of mortality but not sensitive in predicting the neurological outcome. Chorioamnionitis and maternal infections have been shown to be risk factors for HIE and CP. PVL is the strongest and most independent risk factor for the development of CP. Ultrasonographic abnormalities of persistent ventricular enlargement or persistent parenchymal echodensities carry a 50% risk for CP, and large bilateral periventricular cysts carry a risk of 85%. In another study, CP occurred in 56% of infants with PVL and IVH.

3- Classification of Motor Dysfunction

CP can be classified according to the topographic distribution of motor involvement. Motor deficits include monoplegia, diplegia, hemiplegia, triplegia, quadriplegia, and double hemiplegia. Diplegia is present when the lower extremities are primarily affected, although the upper extremities are not completely spared. Spastic diplegia is the most common type of CP and is associated with prematurity. The periventricular germinal matrix, which is a region of active neuronal proliferation, is particularly susceptible to bleeding and hypoxic ischemic injury. The surrounding periventricular white matter contains pyramidal fibers that descend through the internal capsule to supply the lower limbs. More peripheral in the periventricular white matter are the pyramidal tracts of the upper limbs. Therefore, periventricular insult in preterm infants affects the lower limbs more than the upper limbs resulting in spastic diplegia. Note that the term paraplegia should not be used in this context as it implies spinal cord insult involving the lower limbs only *i.e.* not cerebral in origin with completely normal arm function. Hemiplegia is characterized by involvement of one side of the body, with the arm typically more affected than the leg. This is because of larger cortical representation (motor homonculus) of the hand and arm compared to a smaller leg area. Monoplegia refers to single limb involvement. This is usually the result of very mild hemiplegia with arm deficits only. When all four limbs are involved, quadriplegia is the appropriate descriptive term. This is the most disabling with 25% of the affected children requiring total care. Double hemiplegia refers to the child with quadriplegia involving the arms more than the legs with side asymmetry. Triplegia is less common and results from milder and asymmetric double hemiplegia (sparing one leg) or milder asymmetric diplegia (sparing one arm).

ASSOCIATE MANIFESTATIONS &COMPLICATIONS

1- Mental Retardation

Not all children with CP are cognitively impaired. In fact, the commonest type (spastic diplegic CP) is characterized by normal cognition because the lesion is in the periventricular white matter, *i.e.* sparing the cortical grey matter. However, there is a relationship between the severity of CP and mental retardation. Children with spastic quadriplegic CP have greater degrees of mental retardation than children with spastic hemiplegia. Other factors associated with increased cognitive impairment include epilepsy and cortical abnormalities on neuroimaging.

2- Epilepsy

Up to 36% of children with CP have epilepsy, with onset in the first year of life in 70%. Focal seizures with or without secondary generalization are most common with frequently focal EEG abnormalities. Every effort should be made to avoid sedation prior to EEG as this may affect the result of the test. Epilepsy can be an indicator of the severity of neurological injury (quadriplegic CP) or cortical insult (hemiplegic CP). Children with spastic diplegic CP are at a lower risk for epilepsy mainly because their pathology predominantly involves the periventricular white matter. Several new antiepileptic drugs have improved our ability to control the seizures in these children.

3- Feeding, Nutrition, and Growth

These are the most common issues encountered in children with severe CP. About 30% are undernourished, and many show reduced linear growth below the 3rd percentile. Although growth delays appear to be multifactorial in origin, the leading cause appears to be poor nutrition secondary to pseudobulbar palsy. This is an upper motor neuron disorder resulting in poor coordination of sucking, chewing, and swallowing. As well, gastroesophageal (GE) reflux results in regurgitation, vomiting, and possible aspiration. GE reflux can be a source of pain and food refusals in the difficult-to-feed child. Dystonic dyspepsia (Sandifer's syndrome) in children with severe GE reflux can be confused with tonic seizures. Early nasogastric (NG) or gastrostomy tube (GT) feedings can be solutions to these problems with improved growth and greater family satisfaction. NG tube feeding can be used for short-term nutritional support. However, on long-term basis, NG feeding is not socially acceptable and can be associated with nasal discomfort, sinusitis, irritation of the larynx, and recurrent tube blockage or displacement. Surgically or endoscopically placed GT provides a long-term solution to the feeding disorder in conjunction with treating the associated GE reflux. Fundoplication may be indicated at the time of GT placement if medical treatment for GE reflux fails.

4- Bladder Dysfunction

Children with CP are at increased risk for urinary incontinence, urgency, and infections. Spastic CP can be associated with spasticity of the detrusor muscles resulting in small frequent voids and a low capacity irritable bladder. Primary incontinence has been reported in up to 23% of these children and correlates with lower cognition and severe motor deficits. The communication skills and physical ability to go to the bathroom promptly and manage clothing influences the attainment of continence. Adapted toilet seats, handrails, and clothing modifications can increase toileting successes.

5- Bowel Dysfunction

Constipation is common in children with CP and results from multiple factors including poor feeding, reduced water intake, and immobility. Long-term solution involves increased consumption of water, juices, fruits, and vegetables. Initiate bowel evacuation is recommended requiring a combination of laxatives (upper intestinal tract) and enemas or suppositories (lower tract). Afterward, a schedule of softening agents such as artificial powdered fiber or docusate sodium with dietary modifications can result in more regular and softer bowel movements. Sitting on the toilet daily after the main meal takes advantage of the gastro-colic reflex and may be further stimulated occasionally with glycerin suppositories. With effective bowel management programs, many children can attain reasonably regular bowel movements.

6- Sleep Disturbances

Sleep disorders are common in children with CP, particularly those with visual impairment occurring in up to 50% of cases. These children often have disturbed sleep patterns with fragmented sleep and frequent nocturnal awakenings, which is highly disruptive to the parents. Medications that improve the sleep-wake cycle may also decrease spasticity and improve daytime behavior. Hypnotics are generally effective for short periods but loose their effect in few days due to tolerance. Melatonin is a recently developed natural compound with a phase setting effect on sleep. It is the detection of darkness by visual receptors that derives the hypothalamus to stimulate the pineal gland *via* sympathetic pathways to increase melatonin secretion. Visual impairment diminishes the ability of the child to perceive and interpret the multitude of cues for synchronizing their sleep with the environment. This makes these children susceptible to circadian sleep-wake cycle disturbances. Up to 80% of children had dramatic response to a 3 mg melatonin dose at bedtime with reduction in delayed sleep onset, nocturnal awakening, and early arousals. The drug has minimal side effects and no tolerance or dependence.

7- Drooling

Drooling occurs in up to 30% of children with CP. Drooling is usually secondary to mouth opening and/or swallowing difficulties due to pseudobulbar palsy. It is not socially acceptable and can lead to aspiration, skin irritation, and articulation difficulties. Management to this difficult problem is not very effective. Anticholinergic medications, such as Glycopyrrolate, decrease salivation by blocking parasympathetic innervation. Side effects include irritability, sedation, blurred vision, and constipation. Scopolamine is another anticholinergic agent that is available as a skin patch. Surgical re-routing of salivary ducts is an option; however, it may lead to increased aspiration. Recent studies suggest that botulinum toxin injection into the parotid and submandibular glands may be an effective in reducing excessive drooling.

8- Hearing Loss

Certain etiologies increase the risk for hearing loss such as kernicterus, post-meningitis, and congenital rubella. If not diagnosed and treated early, it can interfere with developmental progress and rehabilitation, thereby contributing further to developmental delays. Screening is recommended including behavioral audiometry, auditory-evoked brainstem responses (ABR), or transient evoked otoacoustic emissions. ABR should be performed before or shortly after discharge from the neonatal intensive care unit for every preterm. Hearing assessment is recommended routinely for any child with global developmental delay, particularly if language delay is present. The yield may reach 91% if hearing loss was suspected clinically.

9- Visual Abnormalities

Children with CP are also at increased risk for visual impairment, particularly preterm infants including retinopathy of prematurity, myopia, strabismus, glaucoma, and amblyopia. If not diagnosed and managed early, visual deficits can interfere with developmental progress and rehabilitation. Strabismus can lead to permanent monocular vision loss (amblyopia). Visual impairments can be cortical due to damage to the visual cortex of the occipital lobes. Screening is recommended including acuity, eye movements, and fundoscopy. Visually evoked potentials assess the integrity of the visual pathway from the optic nerve to the visual cortex. Serial ophthalmologic assessments are recommended routinely on any child with global developmental delay, particularly if vision loss is suspected. The yield is 13-25% for refractive errors and strabismus, and 20-50% for visual impairment.

10- Orthopedic Abnormalities

The developing bones grow in the direction of the forces placed upon them. Spasticity can lead to progressive joint contractures, shortened muscles, and hip or foot deformities. Other orthopedic complications that need to be watched for include scoliosis and fractures due to osteomalacia or osteoporosis. These manifestations are more common with severe motor disability and immobility, such as quadriplegia.

DIAGNOSIS

Diagnostic labels should not be taken for granted as misdiagnoses are not uncommon. Many times the term CP is loosely applied to children with various chronic neurological disorders. A comprehensive history for risk factors and genetic background, complete physical and neurological examinations are the mandatory for accurate diagnosis. Serial developmental evaluations may be necessary in the young child for proper diagnosis and follow up. Perinatal complications such as prematurity, head injury, kernicterus, and meningitis are important risk factors for CP. On the other hand, family history of neurological disorders and early or unexplained deaths indicates an undiagnosed inherited neurodegenerative disorder. Familial CP is a misdiagnosis that should not be made. Occasionally CP recurrence occurs due to similar perinatal risk factors; however, family history of CP should always raise the suspicion of an undiagnosed NDD or metabolic disorder. An example is glutaric aciduria type 1, which is an autosomal recessive disorder that results in a clinical picture similar to dyskinetic CP. Another rare disorder that can be confused with CP is dopa responsive dystonia (Segawa disease). In one series, up to 24% of patients with dopa-responsive dystonia had been misdiagnosed as CP. Dystonic movements do not usually cause the wasting, contractures, and deformities that develop in spasticity. Patients usually have a good muscle bulk because of the repeated dystonic contractions. The clue to the diagnosis of dopa-responsive dystonia is the diurnal fluctuation with worsening of symptoms towards the end of the day, and lower limb onset. It is important to recognize this disorder because it responds dramatically to small dose L-dopa. Early warning signs of CP include developmental delay, toe walking, persistent fisting, microcephaly, epilepsy, irritability, poor suck, handedness before 2 years of age (indicating hemiparesis), and scissoring of the lower limbs. In addition, persistence of primitive reflexes can be an early indicator. A multidisciplinary evaluation is recommended and may necessitate input from physiotherapy, occupational therapy, ophthalmology, audiology, orthopedics, radiology, neurology, genetics, developmental pediatrics, and social services. Metabolic and chromosomal analyses are not recommended routinely and indicated if the child has dysmorphic features, family history of delay, or consanguinity. Brain CT may be abnormal in 63-73% of CP cases. Brain MRI is more sensitive than CT, particularly in delineating the extent of white matter changes (Fig. 1). If available, it should be obtained in preference to CT. Once the diagnosis of CP is established, communicating such news to the parents is often both difficult and emotionally unwelcome. As well, most physicians do not feel comfortable dealing with children with neurological disorders such as CP. At the same time, it is important that the transfer of such information is done well as the manner in which neurological bad news is conveyed to parents can significantly influence their emotions, beliefs, and attitudes towards the child, the medical staff, and the future. Most families find the attitude of the news giver, combined with the clarity of the message and the news giver's knowledge to answer questions as the most important aspects of giving the news.

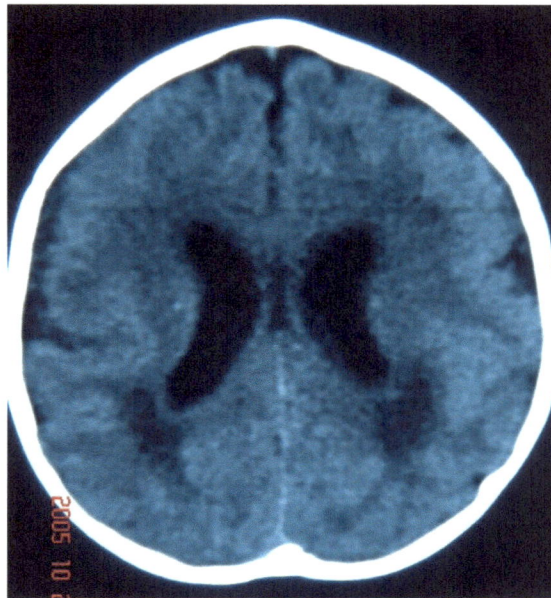

Figure 1: Brain CT showing mild ventricular dilatation with periventricular white matter abnormalities characteristically seen in preterm infants with spastic diplegic cerebral palsy.

MANAGEMENT

The primary care physician should provide anticipatory guidance, immunizations, and developmental surveillance. Additionally, the child's respiratory status should be carefully assessed, as bronchopulmonary dysplasia, reactive airway disease, aspiration, and recurrent chest infections are not uncommon. All routine immunizations should be provided including pertussis vaccine, even if the child has epilepsy. DT, rather than DPT, vaccine is recommended in patients with uncontrolled epilepsy to avoid seizure provocation. Annual influenza vaccination should be provided for those with recurrent or chronic respiratory illnesses. Pneumococcal immunization is recommended for those with chronic or recurrent pulmonary illnesses, and for those at risk for infection with antibiotic resistant organisms, such as children in long-term care facilities and residential settings. Specific treatment options for children with CP include physical and occupational therapy, drug treatments for spasticity (local – intrathecal - systemic), orthopedic and neurosurgical interventions. Most patients require combinations of these therapies; however, physical therapy is always essential. Early institution of physical, occupational, and speech therapies are essential for proper developmental progress. Therapeutic challenges include formulating an individualized treatment plan that is functional goal oriented, time limited, and cost effective. This treatment plan should be team delivered and hospital, home, and/or rehabilitation center based according to the needs of each child. The basic treatment goals include parent education, facilitation of normal motor development and function, prevention of secondary complications such as deformities and disabilities, and improvement of functional acquisition, community integration, and family adjustment. Thus, emphasis has shifted from a strict focus on impairments to a broader focus on function of the child. The key participants on any multidisciplinary treatment team are the child and family as well as physical, and occupational therapists. Physical therapists focus on gross motor skills, including sitting, standing, walking, wheelchair mobility, transfers, and community mobility. Wheelchairs can allow the children to keep up with peers in social, educational, and recreational activities and to develop independence. Power wheelchairs are appropriate for children who lack the strength or coordination to operate a manual chair but demonstrate the cognitive skills necessary for safe navigation. Occupational therapists address the visual and fine motor skills that enable coordinated functions of activities of daily living such as dressing, toileting, eating, bathing, and writing. Forced use or constraint-induced movement therapy can be an effective technique to increase the use of the affected arm in hemiplegic CP. Restraining the stronger arm forces the weaker arm to become more functional. Orthotic interventions are aimed at the prevention and/or correction of deformities, provision of support, facilitation of skill development, and improvement of gait. The most common orthoses used is ankle-foot orthoses (AFO), designed to hold the heel and forefoot in optimal biomechanical position. The multidisciplinary team also includes subspecialists, social workers, nutritionists, and educators, as indicated by the individual needs of the children and their families. This team setting allows for the most effective care delivery system. There are a number of therapeutic interventions that have no scientific literature supporting their use in CP including patterning, conductive education, and hyperbaric oxygen therapy. It is important to emphasize that each child with CP should have the right for comprehensive management, medical education, and environmental modifications that would improve their quality of life.

MANAGEMENT OF SPASTICITY

Spasticity often generates widespread and debilitating consequences for many children with CP including pain, spasm and subsequent contractures. While spasticity need not be treated in every case, physicians today have a wide variety of treatment options. However, tone reduction is indicated only if spasticity interferes with some level of function, positioning, care or comfort. Familiarity with the strengths and weaknesses of each treatment option is an important aspect of clinical decision-making. The impact of spasticity on function must be assessed as children may rely on lower limb extensor tone for stance and ambulation. Spasticity management therefore must be goal-specific, such as to assist with mobility, reduce or prevent contractures, improve positioning and hygiene, and provide comfort. Each member of the child's multidisciplinary team, including the parents, should participate in treatment planning and serial evaluations. In some centers, spasticity clinics exist where a pediatric neurologist, clinical neurophysiologist, orthopedic surgeon, physiotherapist, and occupational therapist assess each child. Team assessment identifies each child's strengths and deficits, set the goals with the family, and develop a comprehensive problem list.

Systemic treatments for spasticity include baclofen, diazepam, dantrolene, and tizanidine, alone or in combinations. Baclofen is the most commonly used oral medication in children with generalized spasticity. Spasticity results from an inadequate release of gamma-aminobutyric acid (GABA), an inhibitory neurotransmitter in the central nervous system. Baclofen is a structural GABA analog enhancing presynaptic inhibition. It crosses the blood-brain barrier poorly. Therefore, high doses may be necessary to achieve clinical response. Side effects include fatigue, irritability, hypotension, drooling, impaired memory and attention, and lowered seizure threshold. Slow drug titration may minimize these side effects. Abrupt withdrawal of baclofen results in rebound spasticity, irritability, and subsequently fever, hallucinations, and seizures. Benzodiazepines, including diazepam, clonazepam, and clobazam, are also useful for generalized spasticity. They increase presynaptic neuronal inhibition through GABA pathways. Sedation and tolerance are the most common adverse effects. Dantrolene exerts its action directly at the muscular level by inhibiting calcium release from sarcoplasmic reticulum and thereby uncoupling excitation and contraction. Muscle weakness, hepatotoxicity, and fatigue are the main side effects making it a less favorable option. Tizanidine is an alpha-2 adrenergic agonist that hyperpolarizes motor neurons and decreases the release of excitatory amino acids. Side effects include nausea, vomiting, hypotension, sedation, and hepatotoxicity. Children with spasticity that are refractory or intolerant to oral medications may be candidates for intrathecal baclofen therapy. After a favorable response to an initial intrathecal test dose, baclofen is provided *via* a programmable, refillable pump, surgically implanted into a subcutaneous abdominal pocket. The pump is connected to a catheter system that delivers a continuous infusion of baclofen into the spinal canal with significant reduction in limb tone. Complications are related to the medication or mechanical pump failure. Overdose typically caused by programming errors, leads to somnolence, hypotonia, and respiratory depression and may progress to loss of consciousness and respiratory failure. Withdrawal can be life threatening, with severe hypertonicity progressing to seizures, hyperthermia, rhabdomyolysis, and multiorgan failure.

Spasticity can be focal, or unequally distributed in the extremities. In such instances, botulinum toxin injections can be used before any surgical considerations. Botulinum toxin blocks the release of acetycholine at the neuromuscular junction with an onset of action of 3-10 days and an average therapeutic duration of 3-6 months. With ongoing active physiotherapy, longer benefits from the injections can occur. Side effects are rare and include transient local pain, fever, and muscle weakness. The drug is not useful if fixed contractures are present. Orthopedic procedures are best left as a last resort for children with severe spasticity and/or fixed contractures or deformities. Tendon lengthening procedures are used to reduce abnormal muscle activity. The timing of these procedures is critical and best planned after the development of a mature gait pattern (5-8 years of age). Rapid growth, postural maturation, and physiologic ligamentous tightening during the first few years of life contraindicate these procedures in the younger child. A lengthened muscle is also weakened, and postoperative rehabilitation is essential. Selective dorsal rhizotomy is a neurosurgical procedure that reduces lower limb spasticity. It involves intraoperative electromyographic monitoring to identify the sensory rootlets from L2 to S2, which, when stimulated, result in abnormal motor responses. Approximately 50% of the stimulated rootlets are cut. The ideal candidate for this procedure is the cooperative, motivated child with spastic diplegic CP who demonstrates good strength, balance, and range of motion in the lower limbs. The procedure reduces lower limb spasticity and improves joint range of motion, and gait.

PROGNOSIS

In general, children have an enhanced capacity for brain plasticity resulting in their capacity to recover and improve from brain insults. There are many possible theories and mechanisms for this brain plasticity. In simple terms, it implies that normal and less damaged areas of the brain have the ability to develop and mature with time to result in developmental progression and motor improvements. A common question asked by the parents is whether the child will be able to walk independently. The ability to sit independently at 2 years of age is predictive of future ambulation. Most children with hemiplegic CP will be able to ambulate independently. Regarding the life expectancy and mortality rates in children with CP, the type and severity of disability, and feeding skills are major determinant. Those who require NG feeding during the first year of life have 5-times greater mortality rate than children with oral feeding. Overall, the probability of reaching age 20 years in a child with severe CP is 50%. Respiratory infections, aspiration, and epilepsy are leading causes of death. Newer therapeutic advances and the degree of parental care have strong influence on the length of survival of these children.

BIBLIOGRAPHY

Jan MMS: Cerebral palsy: Comprehensive Review and Update. Ann Saudi Med 2006;26(2):123-32.

Jan MMS: The Hypotonic Infant: Clinical Approach. J Pediatr Neurol 2007;5(3):181-7.

Jan MM: Misdiagnoses in Children with Dopa-responsive Dystonia. Ped Neurol 2004;31(4):298-303.

Jan MM: Melatonin for the Treatment of Handicapped Children with Severe Sleep Disorder. Ped Neurol 2000;23(3):229-32.

CHAPTER 7

Neurodegenerative Disorders

Abstract: The evaluation of children with suspected neurodegenerative disorders (NDD) requires good background knowledge, accurate assessment, and formulation of a list of differential diagnoses. The initial clinical assessment would guide the physician in requesting the required laboratory investigations in order to reach a specific diagnosis. Reaching a specific diagnosis is of clear importance for providing appropriate therapy, prognosis, and genetic counselling. Many students, residents, and fellows consider neurological disorders, particularly NDD, difficult to master. This reflects the diversity and complexity of various neurological disorders. Different classification systems exist making these disorders confusing to most physicians. However, in this chapter a concise and simple outline with practical tips to facilitate the diagnosis of various NDD will be presented. Important diagnostic tips and possible pitfalls will be discussed, as well as updates in terms of the diagnostic and therapeutic interventions.

Keywords: Degenerative, Metabolic, Motor, Development, Regression, White matter, Grey matter, Leukodystrophy, Mitochondria, Lysosomal.

INITIAL EVALUATION OF SUSPECTED NDD

The evaluation of children with suspected NDD starts with comprehensive history taking followed by detailed physical examination. Diagnostic labels should not be taken for granted, as misdiagnosis is not uncommon. This is particularly true for cerebral palsy, a term loosely applied to children with various chronic neurological disorders. We frequently encounter children diagnosed with cerebral palsy who end up having a progressive CNS disorder. After taking the history and examining the child, formulation of a list of differential diagnoses is an essential first step in formulating a diagnostic hypothesis that directs further laboratory investigations. A list of important NDD and their inheritance patterns is shown in Tables **1** and **2**.

Table 1: Groups of NDD and their inheritance patterns.

Neurodegenerative Disorders (NDD)	Inheritance
Disorders predominantly involving the white matter	
- Canavan Disease	Autosomal recessive
- Alexander Disease	Sporadic
- Krabbe Leukodystrophy	Autosomal recessive
- Metachromatic Leukodystrophy	Autosomal recessive
- Pelizaeus Merzbacher Disease	X linked Recessive
- Adrenoleukodystrophy	X linked recessive
- Multiple Sclerosis	Sporadic
Disorders predominantly involving the Gray matter	
- Menkes Kinky Hair Syndrome	X linked Recessive
- Symptomatic Progressive Myoclonic Epilepsies	Autosomal recessive
(*e.g.* Unverricht-Lundborg disease, lafora disease)	Autosomal recessive
- Progressive Infantile Poliodystrophy	Autosomal recessive
- Sialidosis (Type I)	Autosomal recessive
- Neuronal Ceroid Lipofuscinosis	Variable
- Mitochondrial Encephalopathies	

Table 2: Neurodegenerative disorders with preferential CNS involvement.

Neurodegenerative Disorders	Inheritance
Disorders predominantly involving the basal ganglia	
Juvenile Huntington disease	Autosomal dominant
Dystonia Musculorum Deformans	Autosomal dominant
Hallervorden Spatz Disease	Autosomal recessive
Wilson Disease	Autosomal recessive
Spinocerebellar degeneration and related conditions	
Friedreich Ataxia	Autosomal recessive
Spinocerebellar Ataxia	Autosomal dominant
Olivopontocerebellar Atrophy	Autosomal dominant
Roussy Levy Disease	Autosomal recessive
Spastic paraplegia	
- Familial Spastic Paraplegia	Autosomal dominant
Peripheral neuropathy	
Spinal Muscular Atrophy	Autosomal recessive Autosomal
Infantile Neuroaxonal Dystrophy	recessive Autosomal dominant
Charcot Marie Tooth Disease	Autosomal recessive
Refsum Disease	

These disorders may have predominant white matter involvement (central and/or peripheral demylination) or gray matter involvement (neuronal loss or dysfunction). Important differentiating features between the two groups are summarized in Table 3. Although clinically useful, this distinction is somewhat arbitrary as many NDD have a mixed white and gray matter involvement particularly in the later stages of the disease, *i.e.* secondary demylination following progressive neuronal loss and secondary neuronal loss following progressive demylination. As well, classification schemes are changing with the recent advances at the molecular and cellular levels. Most NDD are now regrouped under specific disease categories according to the defected cellular component. Examples include Peroxisomal disorders (Adrenoleukodystrophy, Zellweger syndrome, Refsum disease), Lysosomal disorders (Krabbe leukodystrophy, Metachromatic leukodystrophy), and Mitochondrial disorders (MELAS, Kearns-Sayre syndrome). However, the distinction between predominantly gray an white matter NDD remain clinically useful in narrowing the differential diagnosis list, examining for associated and complicating features, and guiding the initial laboratory investigations (Table 3).

Table 3: Differentiation between White and Gray matter NDD.

Features	White matter disorders	Gray matter disorders
Age of onset	Usually late (childhood)	Usually early (infancy)
Head size	May have megalencephaly	Usually microcephaly
Seizures	Late, rare	Early, severe
Cognitive functions	Initially normal	Progressive dementia
Peripheral Neuropathy	Early, demylination	Late, axonal loss
Spasticity	Early, severe	Later, progressive
Reflexes	Absent (neuropathy) Exaggerated (long tracts)	Normal or exaggerated
Cerebellar signs	Early, prominent	Late
Fundal examination	May show optic atrophy	Retinal degeneration
EEG	Diffuse delta slowing	Epileptiform spikes
Electromyography (EMG)	Slowed nerve conduction velocity	Usually normal
Evoked potentials (VEP, ABR)	Prolonged or absent	Usually normal
Electroretinograms (ERG)	Normal	Abnormal

HISTORY TAKING

Findings supporting the diagnosis of NDD include an uneventful pregnancy and delivery of a normal full term infant. Postnatal complications such as kernicterus, meningitis, and head trauma should be excluded. Family history of neurological disorders and early or unexplained deaths may indicate an undiagnosed inherited NDD. The nature of the neurological manifestations should be clarified. Detailed developmental history is needed. The distinction between static (non-progressive) and progressive clinical course is very important. Classically, loss of previously acquired milestones (regression) marks the onset of most NDD with subsequent progressive neurological deterioration. However, some NDD or metabolic disorders have a slow rate of progression and can be misdiagnosed as cerebral palsy. Therefore, clear developmental regression may not be evident, particularly in the early stages of the disease or at a younger age of onset. Beware that the neurological consequences of fixed congenital lesions or insults may be delayed for several months because of the immaturity of the nervous system.

Developmental regression does not occur solely in children with genuine NDD. Behavioral syndromes (attention deficit hyperactivity disorder (ADHD), autism, and pervasive developmental disorders) may result in developmental regression, simulating NDD. Other neuropsychiatric disorders such as depression and child neglect may also result in developmental regression. Finally, visual impairment, hearing loss, and intractable epilepsy may interfere with the ability of the child to perceive and utilize the multitude of environmental inputs necessary for normal development, resulting in failure of developmental progression and achievement of milestones (*e.g.* speech, motor, and cognitive arrest). Therefore, a thorough history is very important for the proper assessment of any child with developmental regression and exclusion of other disorders that may simulate NDD. It is needless to say that the approach, management, and prognosis of these disorders are completely different.

CLINICAL EXAMINATION

The neurological examination may be normal in the early stages of some NDD. Behavioral symptoms (*e.g.* ADHD) may be the initial manifestation of certain NDD, specifically metachromatic leukodystrophy, juvenile adrenoleukodystrophy, and subacute sclerosing panencephalitis (SSPE), but will all eventually manifest clinical signs with careful follow up. Careful neurological examination should be performed in any child with behavioral problems to detect early neurological signs. The main differentiating features of predominantly white or gray matter NDD are summarized in Table **3**. The head circumference should be measured and plotted on age appropriate percentile charts. Megalencephaly is an important feature of certain white matter disorders (*e.g.* Canavan and Alexander disease). Microcephaly is a usual feature of many gray matter disorders due to progressive neuronal loss. Examination of the skin and hair can be of diagnostic value in certain metabolic disorders such as Hartnup disease (pellagra-like skin rash) and Menkes disease (kinky hair or pili torti under the microscope). The skin and nervous system have the same embryological origin (ectoderm). Therefore, developmental CNS disorders may have associated skin signs such as neurocutaneous disorders. Some of these disorders may result in progressive loss of CNS function (*e.g.* Sturge Weber syndrome). Examination of the spine for deformities, particularly scoliosis, is important to exclude these commonly associated complications. Examination for dysmorphic features is needed, as some NDD may have associated facial dysmorphism (*e.g.* Zellweger syndrome, Neonatal Adrenoleukodystrophy). Gargoyle-like facial features are characteristic of mucopolysaccharidosis and oligosaccharidosis. Careful and detailed neurological examination is needed in all children with suspected NDD. Examination of eyes may give important diagnostic information as shown in Table **4**. In general, white matter disorders may result in optic atrophy (demylination) while gray matter disorders may result in retinal degeneration, as retinal receptors are in fact neuronal cells. As well, characteristic findings of some neurocutaneous syndromes (*e.g.* lisch nodules), may be seen. Other system examination may provide important clues to the diagnosis. Hepatomegaly and/or splenomegaly are evident in the neurovisceral sphingolipidosis, mucopolysaccharidosis, peroxisomal, and mitochondrial disorders. Cardiopathy occurs in mitochondrial disorders, friedreich ataxia, and mucopolysaccharidosis. Features of progressive renal failure are evident in fabry disease, sialidosis II, and Lowe syndrome.

Table 4: Specific ocular abnormalities in different NDD.

Disorder	Ocular abnormalities
Peroxisomal disorders	Optic atrophy
GM1, GM2, Niemann-Pick Leukodystrophies	Cherry red spot
Mitochondrial disorders Mucopolysaccharidosis	Optic atrophy
Mucolipidosis	Pigmentary retinal degeneration
Ataxia-telangiectasia	Corneal clouding
Cockayne syndrome	Corneal clouding
Wilson disease	Conjunctival telangiectasia
Niemann-Pick disease	Lenticular opacities (cataracts)
Kearns-Sayre syndrome	Kayser-Fleisher corneal ring
Pelizaeus-Merzbacher disease	Vertical gaze palsy
	Progressive external opthalmoplegia Pendular nystagmus

INVESTIGATIONS

Investigations of children with NDD are directed towards identifying the underlying diagnosis and examining associated complications (*e.g.* seizures) as shown in Tables **3** and **5**. The findings on history and physical examination will guide the physician in selecting the required laboratory investigations. Basic blood works may prove useful in certain disorders. Complete blood count may reveal pancytopenia in certain organic acidopathies (*e.g.* isovaleric, proprionic, and methylmalonic acidemias). Blood film may show vacuolated lymphocytes in neuronal ceroid lipofuscinosis, fucosidosis, and sialidosis. Acanthocytosis are characteristic of choreoacanthocytosis, abetalipoproteinemia, and hallervorden-spatz disease. Blood gas analysis will detect metabolic acidosis in many metabolic disorders such as organic acidopathies, urea cycle disorders, and mitochondrial encephalopathies. Serum electrolyte abnormalities may result from adrenal insufficiency in adrenoleukodystrophy. Liver function tests are disturbed in neurovisceral sphingolipidosis and certain gray matter NDD (*e.g.* progressive infantile poliodystrophy). Renal function tests and urinalysis may reveal tubular dysfunction (Lowe syndrome, Wilson disease), nephrotic syndrome (storage diseases), or renal failure (fabry disease, sialidosis II, and Lowe syndrome). Chest X-ray may reveal cardiomegaly in early mitochondrial disorders, friedreich ataxia, and mucopolysaccharidosis. EKG could identify conduction abnormalities that may complicate some of these disorders (*e.g.* refsum disease). Skeletal survey may reveal specific bony abnormalities such as dysostosis multiplex in mucopolysaccharidosis. Neuroimaging, particularly brain MRI, is critical in all children with suspected NDD (Figs. **1-3**). Characteristic MRI features are noted in several white and gray matter NDD including; Alexander disease, Leigh disease, and Hallervorden-Spatz disease. Neuroimaging would exclude slow growing brain tumors, which may result in developmental regression simulating NDD. MRI would also identify developmental defects, malformations, and calcifications. Patients with peroxisomal disorders (Zellweger disease) have associated cortical neuronal migration abnormalities and agenesis of corpus callosum. Serum ammonia, lactate, pyruvate, amino acids, and urine for amino acids and organic acids would screen for most amino acid disorders, organic acidopathies, and urea cycle abnormalities.

Frequently, specific diagnostic tests and enzyme assays are needed to reach a definitive diagnosis. These specialized tests are summarized in Table **5**. The physician should be selective and never use routine or screening tests, as most of these tests are quite expensive. They will frequently involve skin fibroblast culture, CSF examination, DNA studies, nerve, or muscle biopsy. Reaching a specific diagnosis is very important for providing appropriate therapy, prognosis, and genetic counseling. When possible, prenatal diagnosis can be offered in subsequent pregnancies. Specific enzyme levels can be measured in cultures of chorionic villus or amniocytes, but may not be entirely reliable. The use of molecular analysis and specific DNA mutations could improve the accuracy of prenatal diagnosis. Recently, magnetic resonance spectroscopy (MRS) was found to be diagnostic showing increased N-acetylaspartic acid and lactate peaks in Canavan disease and mitochondrial cytopathies, respectively.

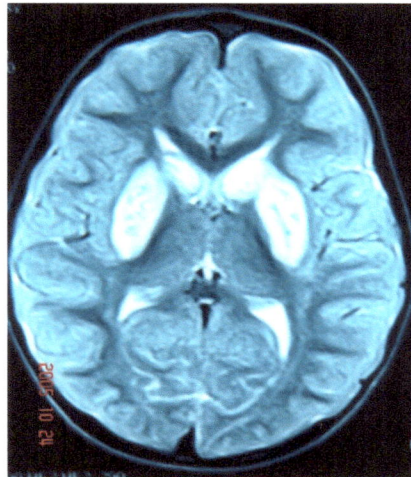

Figure 1: MRI of a child with mitochondrial cytopathy showing abnormal high signal intensity in the region of the basal ganglia.

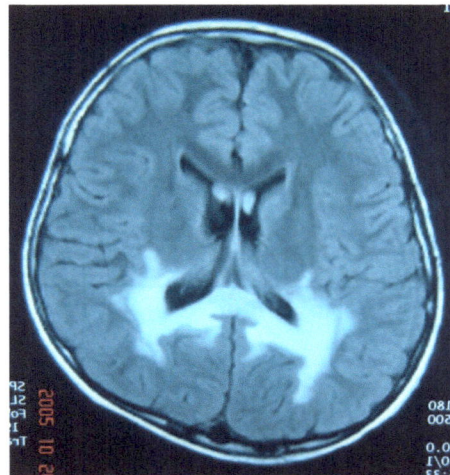

Figure 2: MRI showing early demyelination involving the periventricular region posteriorly in a child with leukodystrophy.

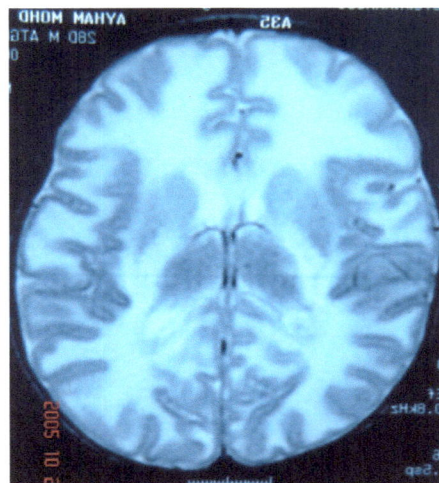

Figure 3: MRI showing more diffuse demyelination in a child with advanced stage of metachromatic leukodystrophy.

Table 5: Specific diagnostic tests of some important NDD.

Neurodegenerative Disorders	Diagnostic Test
Canavan Disease	N-acetylaspartic acid (urine)
Alexander Disease	β-crystallin (CSF)
Krabbe Leukodystrophy	β-galactosidase (leukocytes/fibroblasts)
Metachromatic Leukodystrophy	Arylsulfatase A (leukocytes/fibroblasts)
Adrenoleukodystrophy	Very long chain fatty acids (VLCFA)
Mucopolysaccharidosis Mucolipidosis	Mucopolysaccharides (urine) Oligosaccharides (urine)
Menkes Kinky Hair Syndrome	Serum copper and ceruloplasmin
Lafora disease	Skin biopsy (intracytoplasmic lafora bodies)
Sialidosis (Type I)	α-neuraminidase (leukocytes/fibroblasts)
Neuronal Ceroid Lipofuscinosis	Skin, conjunctival, or rectal biopsy
Mitochondrial Encephalopathies Wilson Disease	Lactate (CSF/blood), Muscle biopsy
Friedreich Ataxia	Urine copper, serum copper & ceruloplasmin
Spinal Muscular Atrophy	DNA studies (blood)
Infantile Neuroaxonal Dystrophy	Muscle biopsy, DNA studies (blood)
Charcot Marie Tooth Disease	Nerve biopsy
Refsum Disease	Nerve biopsy, DNA studies (blood)
Lesch-Nyhan disease	Phytanic acid (blood)
	Hyperuricuria and hyperuricemia

TREATMENT

Treatment of children with NDD is directed towards the underlying disorder, other associated features, and complications. The treatable complications include; epilepsy, sleep disorder, behavioral symptoms, feeding difficulties, gastro-esophageal reflux, spasticity, drooling, skeletal deformities, and recurrent chest infections. These children require a multidisciplinary team approach with the involvement of several specialties including pediatrics, neurology, genetics, orthopedics, physiotherapy, and occupational therapy. Many newer antiepileptic drugs are now available to treat intractable epilepsy. Melatonin, 3 mg at bedtime, has been documented to regulate the sleep-wake cycle, particularly in those with visual impairment. Lioresal or diazepam may relieve spasticity, improve motility of the limbs, and combat pain. Specific treatments to counteract the offending metabolite, replace the dysfunctional enzyme, or vitamin therapy are summarized in Table **6**. Significant advances have been made in regards to specific treatment of NDD. Allogeneic bone marrow transplantation could provide an exogenous source of normal enzymes in several lysosomal storage diseases (Table **6, 7**). Recombinant human α-L-iduronidase has been recently shown to be effective in ameliorating some clinical manifestation of mucopolysaccharidosis. Counseling the families and educating the public about these potentially preventable disorders are very important in the management of these children. Consanguinity needs to be strongly discouraged in order to prevent most NDD in our region.

Table 6: Specific treatments of some important NDD.

Neurodegenerative Disorders	Specific Treatment Modality
Krabbe Leukodystrophy	Bone marrow transplantation
Metachromatic Leukodystrophy	Bone marrow transplantation
Adrenoleukodystrophy	Glyceryl trioleate and trierucate, steroids for adrenal insufficiency, diet low in VLCFA, bone marrow transplantation
Mucopolysaccharidosis	Bone marrow transplantation, recombinant human α-L-iduronidase
Menkes Kinky Hair Syndrome	Copper sulfate
Mitochondrial Encephalopathies	Nicotinamide, riboflavin, dichloroacetate,
Wilson Disease	L-carnitine, CoQ10
Refsum Disease	D-penicillamine, trietine, zinc acetate, liver transplantation
Lesch-Nyhan disease	Reduction of phytanic acid intake
	Allopurinol

BIBLIOGRAPHY

Jan MMS: Approach to Children with Suspected Neurodegenerative Disorders. Neurosciences 2002;7(1):2-6.

Jan MM, Camfield PR: Nova Scotia Niemann-Pick Disease (Type D): Clinical Study of 20 Cases. J Child Neurol 1998;13:75-78.

Kari JA, Alshaya HO, Al-Agah A, Jan MM: Mitochondrial Cytopathy Presenting with Features of Gitelman's Syndrome. Neurosciences 2006;11(2):117-118.

CHAPTER 8

Neurometabolic Disorders

Abstract: Most encephalopaties due to an underlying metabolic (inborn error of metabolism) disorders are genetic, present early in life, and disrupt normal metabolic function. Most these disorders are individually rare, but collectively are common and important cause of preventable morbidity and mortality, both are high if missed or not treated early. There are more than 500 biochemically diverse disorders with many significant recent advances in the diagnosis and treatment that substantially improved prognosis. Pediatricians and neonatologists are vital in early identification, particularly given that the diagnosis needs to be established quickly. Collaboration with a specialized unit is needed for timely consultations and referrals. The neonatal period is a time of substantial catabolism, therefore, neonates has limited response to severe overwhelming illness resulting in death or permanent neurological sequelae. The aim of this chapter is to provide a practical approach to the recognition and investigations of metabolic encephalopathy presenting early in life. Guidelines for the stabilization and initial management will be provided.

Keywords: Metabolic, Motor, Development, Regression, White matter, Grey matter, Mitochondria, Lysosomal, Peroxisomal, Decompensation.

HISTORY

The majority of genetic metabolic disorders are autosomal recessive or occasionally X-linked recessive. Very rarely, autosomal dominant or mitochondrial inheritance is encountered in disorders presenting in the neonatal period. Useful clues include consanguinity, similarly affected sibling, unexplained severe illness in childhood, and undiagnosed neonatal deaths, particularly males on the maternal side. In most cases, both parents are normal (carrying the recessive gene). It is also not unusual that family history is negative and the disorder is secondary to new mutations. Some metabolic encephalopaties may have prenatal presentation. The HELLP syndrome (hyperemesis, liver dysfunction, fatty liver, hemolysis, elevated liver enzymes, low platelets) suggests fatty acid oxidation disorder or long-chain 3-hydroxyacyl coenzyme A dehydrogenase deficiency. Intrauterine seizures (sudden paroxysmal movements) are characteristic of non-ketotic hyperglycinemia or pyridoxine (B6) dependency. As well, certain associated congenital malformations may be detected by prenatal ultrasound.

CLINICAL PRESENTATION

The physician should always maintain high index of suspicion in all ill neonates. The baby may be normal initially until feeding is started. Neonatal sepsis is the most common initial misdiagnosis. It is important to realize that metabolic encephalopathy may coexist with other conditions, such as sepsis. Clinical features are usually subtle in the beginning and proceed to poor feeding, lethargy, poor weight gain, hypotonia, respiratory distress, vomiting, and seizures. The following are the most common presenting features:

1- Acute encephalopathy

2- Liver dysfunction

3- Cardiac disease

4- Seizures

5- Distinctive clinical phenotype

6- Hypotonia

7- Non-immune hydrops fetalis

ACUTE METABOLIC ENCEPHALOPATHY

Acute encephalopathy results from the accumulation of diffusible metabolites or precursor, such as ammonia. This accumulation can be due to deficiency of an essential product (*e.g.* adenosine triphosphate) or defective transport process (*e.g.* carnitine). Most of these metabolites cross the placenta and are cleared by the mother, and affected infants are usually normal at birth. Most of affected babies are born following a normal term pregnancy, with normal birth weight and are well for days or longer depending on the severity of the metabolic block and the environmental triggers. Most infants are re-admitted after discharge from the nursery because of poor feeding, vomiting, lethargy, irritability, or seizures. Tachypnea may indicate metabolic acidosis and cerebral edema frequently leads to relentless deterioration. These neonates may become unresponsive to symptomatic therapy (*e.g.* fluids, ventilation, and antibiotics). Persistent metabolic acidosis with normal tissue perfusion should suggest the diagnosis. Associated hypoglycemia, hyperammonemia, and organic acidosis, should be suspected. Acute metabolic encephalopathy is typical of urea-cycle defects, organic acidemias, and fatty acid oxidation defects. Rarely, some amino acid disorders present in encephalopathy, such as MSUD (sweet urinary odor derives from ketoacids). Baseline investigations in acutely ill neonates with suspected metabolic disorder are summarized in Table **1**.

Table 1: Suggested baseline investigations in acutely ill neonates with suspected metabolic disorder.

URINE	Ketones
	Reducing substances
	Amino acids
	Organic Acids
BLOOD	Blood gases
	Electrolytes (anion gap)
	Glucose, CBC, blood Film
	Liver function test
	Ammonia, Lactate, Pyruvate, Amino acids

LACTIC ACIDOSIS

The presence of lactic acidosis suggest an inherited mitochondrial transport chain or pyruvate metabolism defects, however, poor tissue perfusion due to meningitis or sepsis should be excluded. There is persistent increase in blood lactate with levels >6 mmol/L (normal < 2. 0 mmol/L) and increased anion gap (>20 mEq/L). CSF lactate and pyruvate should be obtained if serum levels are normal. This test should be obtained after excluding brain edema on neuroimaging. Normal blood and CSF lactate excludes most mitochondrial disorders. However, muscle and/or liver biopsies provide tissue for biochemical, ultrastructural and molecular analyses for precise determination of the biochemical and genetic defects. Citric acid cycle, pyruvate dehydrogenase (PDH), and pyruvate carboxylase (PC) defects may also result in lactic acidosis. Citric acid cycle defects can be diagnosed by checking the urine for organic acid. PDH or PC typically results in normal lactate/pyruvate ratio and high citrulline. Specific enzymatic assays are confirmative.

ORGANIC ACIDOSIS

Two important etiologies include propionic acidemia (propionyl-CoA carboxylase deficiency) and methyl-malonic acidemia (L-methylmalonyl-CoA mutase deficiency). Both result in very severe metabolic acidosis due to accumulation of organic acids with increased anion gap (>20 mEq/L). Moderate to severe hyperammonemia and hypoglycemia are usually associated. Pancytopenia indicates secondary bone marrow suppression.

HYPOGLYCEMIA

Hypoglycemia is commonly encountered with prematurity, intrauterine growth retardation, maternal diabetes mellitus, and sepsis. Unexplained, severe and/or persistent hypoglycemia could indicate a metabolic cause. Fasting hypoglycemia requiring >12 µg/kg/min of dextrose suggests hyperinsulinism. Associated metabolic acidosis could indicate organic acidemia or defect in gluconeogenesis such as glycogen storage disease type 1 or fructose 1, 6 biphosphatase deficiency. Associated liver disease indicates galactosemia or hereditary fructose intolerance and ketosis suggests MSUD. Other disorders associated with hypoglycemia include fatty acid oxidation disorders and medium-chain acyl-CoA dehydrogenase deficiency. Both are characterized by fasting hypoglycemia and family history of sudden infant death syndrome (SIDS) or near-miss SIDS. Elevated transaminases, hyperammonemia, and reduced levels of carnitine are characteristic. However the diagnosis is established by the finding of abnormal fatty acid metabolites in urinary organic acid screening, acylglycine analysis, and plasma acylcarnitine analysis.

HYPERAMMONEMIA

Hyperammonemia is usually associated with mild respiratory alkalosis. It is a medical emergency as ammonium is a potent neurotoxin and the duration of hyperammonemic coma correlates with CNS damage. Several metabolic encephalpathies can be responsible including organic acidoses and fatty acid oxidation defects, which results in secondary inhibition of the urea cycle by accumulating metabolites. Transient hyperammonemia of the newborn occurs in the premature babies with lung disease, however a glutamine/ammonium ratio of >1. 6 suggests a urea-cycle defect.

Jaundice and Liver Dysfunction

Several metabolic disorders may present with jaundice, elevated liver enzymes, hepatomegaly, clotting abnormalities and hypoglycemia. These include galactosaemia, tyrosinaemia type I, hereditary fructose intolerance, and mitochondrial disorders. As well, peroxisomal disorders may be associated with jaundice and hepatomegaly. Cystic fibrosis, antitrypsin deficiency, citrullinaemia type II, Nieman Pick type C, inborn errors of bile acid synthesis, haemochromatosis, and congenital disorders of glycosylation, are other examples. Finally, fatty acid oxidation defects can present with hepatomegaly and hypoglycemia.

CARDIAC DISEASE

Long chain fatty acid oxidation disorders can present with cardiomyopathy, arrhythmias and cardiac arrest. Mitochondrial disorders, Barth syndrome, and congenital disorders of glycosylation can be associated with cardiomyopathy. Glycogen storage disease type IV and heart-specific phosphorylase kinase deficiency present with cardiomyopathy or hydrops fetalis. Rarely, cardiomyopathy may be a complication of lysosomal storage disorders.

Encephalopathy with Seizures

Perinatal asphyxia is the commonest cause of neonatal encephalopathy with seizures. In that case, the seizures usually occur early and represent a predominant feature of the encephalopathy. Important metabolic disorders with this presentation include non-ketotic hyperglycinemia (hypotonia, apnea, hiccoughs), pyridoxine dependent epilepsy, folinic acid responsive seizures, and disorders of the glucose transporter. Cysteine, sulphite oxidase, molybdenum cofactor defects present with hypotonia, cerebral calcification, choreo-athetosis, lens dislocation and seizures. In this case, the urine will reveal raised S-sulphocysteine, thiosulphite, and low uric acid

DISORDERS WITH DISTINCTIVE PHENOTYPES

Lysosomal (mucolipodosis, GM1 gangliosidosis) and peroxisomal (Zellweger syndrome) storage disorders frequently have a distinctive phenotype. Congenital disorders of glycosylation and untreated maternal phenylketonuria (PKU) can cause microcephaly and IUGR. Pyruvate dehydrogenase deficiency also has a characteristic facial dysmorphism. As well as, glutaric aciduria type II (facial dysmorphism and hypospadias) and menkes disease (facial dysmorphism and hair fragility).

Severe Hypotonia

Severe hypotonia is seen characteristically in peroxisomal storage disorders (Zelweger), nonketotic hyperglycinemia, congenital lactic acidosis, and congenital disorders of glycosylation (N-linked oligosaccharides defect).

INITIAL ACUTE MANAGEMENT

The acutely ill neonate has to be treated early and aggressively. Eliminate the intake of precursors of toxic metabolites (enteral feeds), but administer enough calories to switch off further catabolism. Intravenous fluids with 10% dextrose should be given with higher than maintenance rates. Avoid fluid overload, and aggressively treat cerebral edema, which is characteristic of MSUD and urea-cycle defects. Additional calories can be given *via* IV intralipid unless a disorder of fatty acid oxidation is suspected. Treat associated complications, such as shock, hypoglycemia, dehydration, electrolyte imbalances, and infection. Hyperammonemia is treated by Na benzoate or sodium phenylbutyrate. Na bicarbonate should be administered if metabolic acidosis is associated with a serum bicarbonate of <15 mEq/L. In severe lactic acidosis, biotin can be given empirically to treat possible multiple carboxylase deficiency. If the metabolic acidosis is unexplained, IM vitamin B12 should be given for possible methylmalonic acidemia. The use of other vitamin cocktails or specific medications should be coordinated by the metabolic team (Table **2**). If the child does not improve and becomes semicomatosed or comatosed, hemodialysis or haemofiltration should be considered. Some patients die despite aggressive therapy and post-mortem examination seldom provides clues to the diagnosis. However, several specimens can be obtained for future assessment if the diagnosis is not clear after death as shown in Table **3**.

Table 2: Vitamin cofactors used for suspected mitochondrial encephalopathies.

Vitamin cofactors	Dose
Biotin	50 mg/day
Thiamine	300 mg/day
Riboflavin	100 mg/day
Coenzyme Q10	4 mg/kg/day (maximum 300 mg/day)
Vitamin K	0.36 mg/kg/day
Vitamin C	57 mg/kg/day (maximum 1.5 g/day)
L-carnitine	100 mg/kg/day

Table 3: Specimens obtained before or within 2-4 hr after death for future examination if no diagnosis was identified.

Filter paper spots (Tandom Mass Spectrometry)
Freeze (-70C) 10 ml of plasma, 5-10 ml of urine, 1 ml of CSF
Skin, liver, muscle biopsy (EM, culture, histopathology, enzymology)

SUMMARY

Metabolic encephalopathy are individually rare disorders, but collectively not uncommon. Most of these genetic disorders with an underlying metabolic etiology are increasing. Pediatricians and neonatologists must be vigilant in early detection as early diagnosis and intervention is crucial to avoid CNS sequelae and death. Collaboration with a specialized unit is needed. Tandom mass spectrometry newborn screening should be highly considered for early identification given the remarkable recent advances in treatment that substantially improved the prognosis of these disorders.

BIBLIOGRAPHY

Jan MMS: Approach to Children with Suspected Neurodegenerative Disorders. Neurosciences 2002;7(1):2-6.

Kari JA, Alshaya HO, Al-Agah A, Jan MM: Mitochondrial Cytopathy Presenting with Features of Gitelman's Syndrome. Neurosciences 2006;11(2):117-8.

CHAPTER 9

Seizures and Epilepsy

Abstract: Seizures are the most common cause of referral to pediatric neurology services and represent an important cause of pediatric morbidity. Epilepsy (recurrent unprovoked seizures) is a common neurological disorder in children with a frequency of 4-8 cases per 1000 children. Seizures in children have wide variations in clinical expression with age specific presentation. For example, primary generalized tonic clonic and absence seizures are extremely uncommon in infants and never occur in neonates. Benign rolandic epilepsy of childhood has an onset at 5 years and usually remits by age 15. Physicians are frequently faced with anxious parents and are required to make rational decisions regarding the workup and management of childhood epilepsy. They are subsequently required to provide counseling and information about the prognoses to the involved families. The aim of this chapter is to provide an updated overview of pediatric epilepsy and review the most recent diagnostic and therapeutic recommendations.

Keywords: Seizure, Epilepsy, Ictus, Aura, Semiology, Conciousness, Awareness, EEG, MRI, Shuddering, Syncope, Antiepileptic drugs.

DEFINITIONS

A seizure (ictus) represents transient neurological manifestations due to an abnormal, excessive neuronal discharges originating from the cerebral cortex. This discharge can result in many different neurological manifestations according to the seizure origin and spread (*e.g.* sensory, motor, somatosensory, psychic). A convulsion refers to a seizure with motor manifestations, usually generalized tonic clonic. A "fit" is a term that should not be used as it may imply a psychogenic etiology. Epilepsy (to be attacked in Greek) is recurrent (2 or more) unprovoked seizures. Transient provoked seizures caused by fever, illness, electrolyte imbalance, toxic exposure, or head injury, are not classified as epilepsy. Epilepsy is not a specific disease, but rather a manifestation of a variety of congenital or acquired brain insults.

CLASSIFICATION

Seizures can be clinical or subclinical (electrographic) with EEG but no clinical manifestations. The International League against Epilepsy (ILAE) classification system is summarized in Table **1**. A partial (focal) seizure can be simple with normal consciousness or complex when consciousness is impaired (not necessarily completely lost). Patients may become confused disoriented or have no memory of a complex partial seizure, however, they always remember a simple attack (aura). Therefore, an aura is a simple partial seizure with clinical manifestations that depends on the involved region of the brain. Partial seizures can be motor (frontal), sensory (parietal), visual (occipital), autonomic or psychic (temporal). An initial simple partial seizure may spread to neighboring or remote brain regions resulting in impaired consciousness (simple to complex) or in a generalized tonic-clonic seizure. This later type is called a secondarily generalized seizure, to differentiate it from seizures that are generalized from the onset (primary generalized). Myoclonic, atonic, and absence seizures are all primary generalized seizures. Note that the majority of generalized tonic clonic seizures in children are secondarily generalized, which has important diagnostic and therapeutic implications. Epilepsy syndromes (Table **1**) are associated with one or more seizure types and other characteristic clinical, EEG, or prognostic characteristics. For example febrile seizures, a common syndrome, is a special (situation related) benign epilepsy syndrome characterized by focal (atypical) or generalized (typical) seizures.

EPIDEMIOLOGY

The overall prevalence of epilepsy ranges between 4-8/1, 000 population. Children <10-years have a lifetime prevalence of 6/1, 000. Up to 5% of children will have a febrile seizure in the first five years of life. Most seizures start at the extremes of age. The incidence is highest in the first year of life and lowest in early and middle adulthood. It begins increasing in the 50s, with a dramatic increase after age 60 when the incidence exceeds that of infancy. Males are at higher risk; however, no significant racial differences exist. Partial seizures are the most common type accounting for more than 50% of all seizures; complex partial seizures being the most common. Up to 12% of epilepsy patients present in status epilepticus. Of the children with epilepsy, 35% had an associated developmental disorder such as mental retardation, cerebral palsy, visual impairment, or hearing impairment.

Table 1: International classification of seizures and epilepsy syndromes.

I. Seizure Classification
1- Partial (focal) seizures
a- Simple (normal consciousness)
b- Complex (disturbed level of consciousness)
c- Simple evolving to complex partial
2- Generalized
a- Primary generalized (generalized from the onset)
b- Secondary generalized (starting as simple or complex partial)
c- Unclassified
II. Classification of Epilepsy Syndromes
1- Localization related (focal)
Idiopathic (*e.g.* benign rolandic epilepsy)
Cryptogenic (*e.g.* non-lesional partial epilepsy)
Symptomatic (*e.g.* mesial temporal sclerosis, glioma)
2- Generalized
Idiopathic (*e.g.* Absence epilepsy)
Cryptogenic (*e.g.* Myoclonic astatic epilepsy)
Symptomatic (Infantile spasms, Lennox Gastaut syndrome)
3- Undetermined (*e.g.* severe myoclonic epilepsy of infancy)
4- Special (situation related such as febrile seizures)

ETIOLOGY

A seizure may be an isolated event with no obvious cause or triggered by acute metabolic disturbances or fever. Epilepsy may be idiopathic (usually genetic), cryptogenic (undiagnosed cause with associated neurological or developmental deficits), or symptomatic (known cause). This etiologic classification also applies to epilepsy syndromes (Table 1). Epilepsy results from an insult to the cerebral cortex, particularly the neocortical gray matter and the limbic system (hippocampus and amygdala). Most patients have no underlying organic pathology. Causes include congenital anomalies, developmental disorders (such as migration defects), vascular, traumatic, hypoxic, infectious, neoplastic, and degenerative disorders. With the advent of neuroimaging, particularly MRI, subtle brain malformations and migration disorders are increasingly recognized. Advances in genetic research also allowed the identification of the chromosomal location and the abnormal gene in familial epilepsy. Mesial temporal sclerosis (MTS) is the most common lesion encountered in patients referred to temporal lobectomy. Patients with MTS often have history of atypical febrile seizures.

SEMIOLOGY

The seizure discribtion including symptoms (history) and signs (observation and video monitoring is termed semiology. This is described in details in the next chapter. Seizures are stereotyped and random events; however, some children have several seizure types. Different seizures may be due to varying cortical involvement or propagation to neighboring cortex. A seizure may be characterized by flashing lights in one visual field (occipital), followed by eye deviation away from the side of onset (spread to association cortex), followed by loss of awareness and automatic behavior (spread to the temporal lobe), and then culminates in a generalized tonic-clonic seizure (secondarily generalized). Facial twitching followed by speech arrest supports the diagnosis of a partial seizure originating from the dominant hemisphere. During complex partial seizures, the patient may have simple oral-buccal automatisms (chewing, swallowing, sucking), or complex motor phenomena (bicycling, flailing, walking). On some occasions, the patient may experience only the first stage of the seizure with absence of the later stages. Only close questioning of the parents and child will uncover this valuable localizing information. We see many children with a referral diagnosis of generalized tonic clonic seizures for whom close questioning yields information that the seizures are focal in origin. Generalized motor seizures cannot be interrupted by vocal or painful stimulation, distinguishing them from non-epileptic events. Atonic seizures (drop attacks) usually occur in neurologically abnormal children with multiple seizure types such as lennox-gastaut syndrome (LGS). Absence seizures (previously called Petit Mal) cannot be interrupted by vocal or tactile stimulation as can the non-epileptic staring spells (day dreaming or inattention) seen in children with attention deficit hyperactivity disorder. Absence seizures are very repetitive and often result in brief interruptions of conversation or physical activity for seconds (usually less than 30 seconds). This helps in distinguishing absence seizures from the staring spells due to complex partial seizures, which are usually less frequent (up to 2-4/day), longer in duration (1-2 minutes), and may be associated with aura, cyanosis, and/or postictal sleep. Children with absence seizures have no memory of the event and no postictal sleep (Table **2**).

Table 2: Differentiating staring due to absence from that of complex partial seizures.

Features	Abscence	Complex Partial
Sleep activation	None	Common
Hyperventilation	Results in seizure induction	No activating effect
Seizure frequency	Frequent, many per day	Less frequent
Seizure onset	Abrupt	Slow
Aura	None	If preceded by a simple partial seizure
Automatism	Rare	Common
Progression	Minimal	Evolution of features
Cyanosis	None	Common
Motor signs	Rare, or minimal	Common
Seizure duration	Brief (usually <30 sec)	Minutes
Postictal confusion or sleep	None	Common
Postictal dysphasia	None	Common in seizures originating from the dominant hemisphere

HISTORY TAKING

Careful and detailed history is the cornerstone of an accurate diagnosis. A timed description of the child's behavior during the event is needed for accurate classification and localization. The first encounter may require follow-up visit or phone call to other witnesses, such as a teacher or an older sister. Asking one of the parents to videotape the event, whenever possible, can be diagnostic. The physician should remember to include the child in the conversation who may provide valuable information. If the description is not clear, the physician can ask the parent to mimic the event, or the physician may mimic different seizures to find a match for the child's events. A previous diagnosis of epilepsy should not be accepted without a confirmatory history. The history of each event should be divided in four stages including preictal, beginning of the seizure, ictal, and postictal phase. In the preictal phase, provoking or precipitating factors should be sought of such as fever, illness, ingestion, compliance, and head injury. The time of the seizure is important as some occur predominantly in sleep (benign rolandic seizures, tonic seizures in LGS, and frontal lobe seizures). History of any brief focal signs or symptoms (aura) at the beginning of the more dramatic seizure should be obtained. Anxious parents tend to describe the most dramatic part of the seizure and ignore the more subtle initial focal symptoms. Aura should not be confused with prodrome, which precedes generalized tonic clonic seizures by several hours to a day. Prodromal symptoms include headache irritability, and personality change, all are rare in children and are not part of the ictus. Tonic seizures immediately preceded by crying or minor trauma should alert the physician to the diagnosis of breath-holding spells. Falls following standing in a stressful situation (classroom) and preceded by dizziness suggests vasovagal syncope. A cardiac cause, such as prolonged QT interval, should be considered if the child is pale during the event. During the seizure, the exact description of the clinical manifestations and their duration is needed. Clusters of tonic spasms upon awakening suggest infantile spasms. A non-epileptic seizure (pseudoseizure) should be suspected if the patient has minimal or no movements during a prolonged unresponsive event. Waxing and waning motor activity with tight eye closure are consistent with a pseudoseizure, particularly if passive eye opening is resisted. Postictal unilateral headache or transient weakness (Todd's paresis) has a lateralizing value indicating a contralateral hemispheric origin. Postictal aphasia (inability to talk despite being able to follow simple commands) suggests a seizure originating from the speech area of the dominant hemisphere. Visual field defects have localizing value indicating occipital lobe origin. Other important aspects of the history include development, past medical, family and social histories. Enquiring about history of meningitis, encephalitis, head injury, and febrile seizures is mandatory in every child with epilepsy. Positive family history of epilepsy or consanguinity should raise the suspicion of an inherited genetic epileptic disorder.

DIFFERENTIAL DIAGNOSES

Many paroxysmal events may simulate epilepsy in the neonatal period, infancy, and childhood. Careful and detailed history is the cornerstone of a correct diagnosis. A timed description of the child's behavior during the event is needed for accurate diagnosis. The first encounter may require follow-up visit or phone call to other witnesses, such as a teacher or an older sister. Asking one of the parents to videotape the event, whenever possible, can be diagnostic. The physician should remember to include the child in the conversation who may provide valuable information. If the description is not clear, the physician can ask the parent to mimic the event, or the physician may mimic different movements to find a match for the child's events. A previous diagnosis of epilepsy should not be accepted without a confirmatory history. The following disorders may be mistaken for epilepsy including benign sleep myoclonus, hyperekplexia, shuddering episodes, night terrors, breath holding spells, dystonic dyspepsia, tics, syncope, and pseudoseizures.

Benign Sleep Myoclonus

Benign sleep myoclonus is a normal phenomenon that occurs in the lighter stages of sleep. It is usually mistaken for seizures by inexperienced parents. It mainly affects neonates and young infants as they fall asleep, usually while feeding in the parents lap. Arm, body, or leg jerking will not stop by restraining the limb. However, they will disappear spontaneously if the baby wakes up or go into deeper stages of sleep. Clinical examination and EEG, if done, are normal. The parents should be reassured and no further intervention is needed.

Hyperekplexia

Hyperekplexia is familial pathological startle response. Body jerk is evoked by auditory or sensory stimuli and may be mistaken for myoclonus. This is unlike jitteriness that is seen in neonates upon handling. Hypertonia, hyperreflexia, apnea, and vomiting may be the presenting features in the neonatal period. The disorder is the result of a dysfunction in cortical inhibitory regulation on the brain stem due to chromosome 5q defect (glycine receptor gene). Beware that auditory myoclonus may be the presenting feature of certain neurometabolic disorders such as Tay Sach's disease. Therefore, careful examination and follow up is needed. Benzodiazepine or phenobarbitone may be used; however, most patients need no treatment with spontaneous improvement as they grow older.

Shuddering Attacks

This is a rare movement that can be confused with epilepsy in young infants. Shoulder shivering occurs during spontaneous activity, such as playing. The child will stop momentarily and have these shoulder shivering movements briefly with no loss of consciousness, cyanosis, or fall. Then, spontaneous activity will resume. If an EEG is done its always normal. No treatment is needed. Family history is usually positive for essential tremor.

Night Terrors

Night terrors usually occur after the first few hours of sleep in a 4-8 years old child. The child wakes up screaming and crying. He will be confused and terrified. He may sit-up and sweat for several minutes. Nothing that the parents do can terminate the episode that usually ends by falling back to sleep. Next day, the child has no memory of the event, which helps in distinguishing these episodes from night mares. Night terror can be related to daytime experiences and frequently associate with sleep walking, however, it is benign and the parents need to be reassured. Light snack, shower, and a relaxing story are usually helpful at bed time.

Breath Holding Spells

Tonic seizures immediately preceded by crying or minor trauma should alert the physician to the diagnosis of breath-holding spells. The child is usually less than 5 years of age. Breathing usually stops on inspiration and the child quickly become cyanosed and limp. During the episodes, the parents should avoid lifting the child to an upright position, which may lead to decreased cerebral perfusion and secondary generalized tonic seizure. Therefore, the child should be always kept flat during these episodes. Breath holding spells are brief, infrequent, and frequently related to iron deficiency (not necessarily iron deficiency anemia). Iron therapy can result in complete resolution, however, behavioral modification is always recommended to prevent special treatment and improper parental overprotection of such a child. Piracetam or levetiracetam can be used for resistant and frequent cases.

Dystonic Dyspepsia (Sandifer syndrome)

Dystonic dyspepsia takes the form of recurrent neck hyperextension and repetitive swallowing movements associated with gastroesophageal reflux. The child looks uncomfortable, but alert. The episodes are related to feeding and frequently associated with recurrent vomiting. Most of these patients have static encephalopathy or cerebral palsy, which make them predisposed to reflux. Many may also have seizures; therefore accurate history will differentiate between these events and seizures.

Tics

Tics are complex stereotyped movements that can be incorporated by the child into normal movements. Vocal tics (throat clearing or coughing) can be associated. There is no disruption in the level of consciousness and the movements can be suppressed by the child, however, they are involuntary. Tics increase with stress and never occur in sleep. If tics are due to Tourette syndrome, associated co-morbidities may include attention deficit hyperactivity disorder, obsessive compulsive behaviour, and learning difficulties. Family history of tics or the other co-morbid conditions is frequently positive.

Syncope

Falls following standing in a stressful situation suggests vasovagal syncope. Syncope (fainting) frequently occurs in older children and adolescents. The child is always in an upright position (sitting or standing) or in a transition from flat to upright position. It can be preceded by dizziness or vision loss (presyncope). The fall is frequently slow, unlike drop attacks, so the child may be able to change position or sit down. The child may be pale, but never cyanosed and is normal afterward. Most often, the child will remember the onset. Complete blood count is recommended to exclude anemia. EKG should be obtained to exclude prolonged QT interval. No specific treatment is needed, however, the child should be instructed to sit or lie down at the onset of symptoms to prevent falls or injury.

Pseudoseizures

A non-epileptic seizure (pseudoseizure) should be suspected if the patient has minimal or no movements during a prolonged unresponsive event. Waxing and waning generalized motor activity with tight eye closure are consistent with a pseudoseizure, particularly if passive eye opening is resisted. A pseudoseizure can be induced by suggestions and may be interrupted by vocal or painful stimulation. Up to 20% of patients with pseudoseizures also have epilepsy. Continuous video-EEG monitoring is usually needed to confirm the diagnosis. Psychosocial triggers are the most common complicating issues.

PHYSICAL EXAMINATION

Anthropometric parameters should be measured and plotted on age appropriate percentile charts. Abnormal head size, weight, and height may be associated with certain disorders and syndromes that may have neurological manifestations. In the acute situation, vital sign measurements are critical. Fever or hypothermia, particularly in infants, may indicate an underlying CNS infection. In patients with disturbed level of consciousness, high blood pressure and bradycardia (Cushing reflex) indicate increased intracranial pressure due to hemorrhage or a space occupying lesion. Examination for meningeal irritation signs is important to exclude raised intracranial pressure. Neck stiffness may indicate meningitis, meningoencephalitis, subarachnoid hemorrhage, or cerebellar herniation. The blood pressure should be measured in the supine and standing positions to assess postural drop in patients with vasovagal syncope. Skin exam is important as the skin and the nervous system have the same embryologic origin (ectoderm). Therefore, developmental CNS disorders may have associated skin signs (neurocutaneous disorders) such as ash leaf spots of tuberous sclerosis, facial angioma of Sturge-Weber syndrome, café-au-lait spots of neurofibromatosis, nevi of the linear nevus syndrome, and swirling hypopigmentation of Ito syndrome (Fig. **1**). Examination of the skull for shape, fontanel size and tenseness, sutures for premature fusion or wide separation are important. As well, skull auscultation for bruits may indicate an underlying arteriovenous malformation. Many syndromes may have associated CNS anomalies or features. It is important therefore to carefully assess the patient for dysmorphic features (face, mouth, palate, hands, and feet). Ophthalmologic examination may provide clues to the child's seizures (leish nodules or retinal hamartomas). Abdominal examination may reveal organomegaly in storage diseases. Cardiac examination is necessary if a cardiogenic cause for the child's episodes is suspected. Careful CNS examination is needed to exclude focal neurological signs. Some seizures can be provoked in the examination room such as absence seizures (hyperventilation) or startle precipitated seizures (auditory stimuli). Hyperventilation is performed by asking the child to blow on a napkin for up to 3 minutes by taking deep breaths. If an absence seizure develops, the examiner should name a color, number, or an object and then ask the child if he or she remembers it afterward (Table **2**).

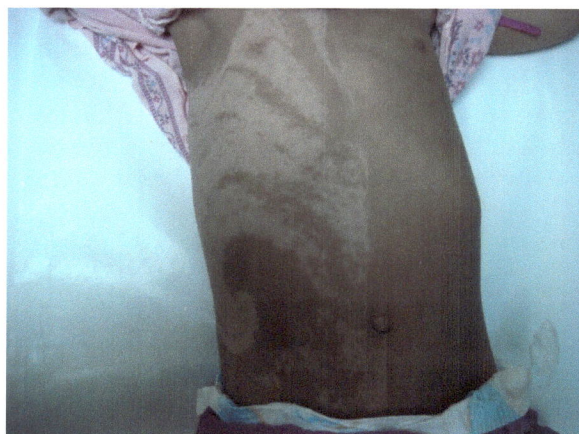

Figure 1: Swirling hypopigmentation of Ito syndrome.

INVESTIGATIONS

Investigations are directed toward confirming the clinical diagnosis, seizure classification, and uncovering the underlying etiology. Extensive diagnostic testing may not be necessary if the history and physical examination provide an obvious etiology for the seizure. Initial laboratory investigations include serum electrolytes, calcium, phosphorous, alkaline phosphatase, magnesium, and glucose. In febrile children, complete blood count and appropriate cultures are indicated; however, meningitis and meningo-encephalitis are the main concern. Seizures can be the presenting, but not the only feature, of up to 15% of children with meningitis. Infants with meningitis may not display meningeal signs, however, they have other symptoms and signs that strongly suggest the diagnosis (*e.g.* altered state of consciousness, persistent vomiting, bulging fontanel, abnormal neurological signs). It is recommended that lumbar puncture (LP) be strongly considered in infants less than 12 months, considered in infants 12-18 months, and if clinically indicated in those greater than 18 months of age. LP should also be strongly considered if the child had received prior oral antibiotics that may mask the clinical manifestations of meningitis or results in transient improvement. Routine LP in all children with febrile convulsions is clearly not warranted. Infants with a history of vomiting, diarrhea, and altered fluid intake should have serum electrolyte profiles to exclude hypernatremia or hyponatremia. Clinical evidence of dehydration and prolonged drowsiness or postictal obtundation are also indications for measurement of serum electrolytes, blood sugar, calcium, and urea nitrogen. If an acute cause cannot be found, the child may be experiencing the initial seizure of an epileptic disorder. EEG and neuroimaging should be considered in these children. Testing for metabolic or genetic disorders should be performed if these disorders were suspected clinically.

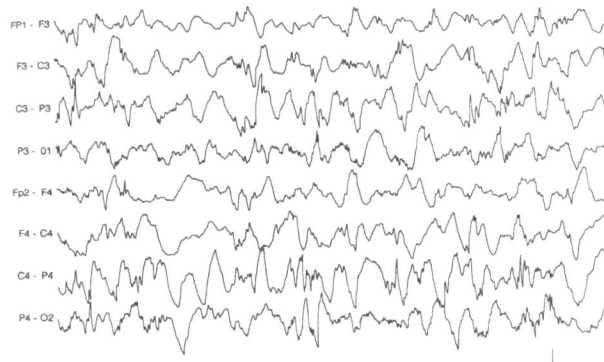

Figure 2: Chaotic EEG of a child with infantile spasms showing the characteristic high voltage slow delta waves and multifocal spikes (Hypsarrhythmia).

ELECTROENCEPHALOGRAPHY (EEG)

EEG is a very important tool in investigating children with epilepsy. Although epilepsy is a clinical diagnosis, accurate EEG interpretation often provides supportive evidence and helps in seizure classification. As well, the EEG shows some characteristic abnormalities in certain epilepsy syndromes, such as Infantile spasms (Fig. **2**), Lennox-Gastaut syndrome, and absence seizures (Fig. **3**). However, note that the EEG does not rule out or diagnose epilepsy. In other words, it only confirms the clinical impression. Some non-epileptic events may simulate epilepsy including breath holding spells, syncope, tics, migraine related phenomena (*e.g.* benign paroxysmal vertigo), and psychogenic seizures. The neurological examination and interictal EEG are usually normal; however, a complete event description accurately identifies the nature of these events. The yield of routine EEG is low in neurologically normal children with febrile seizures even if the seizure is atypical. When the clinical suspicion of epilepsy is high and the awake recorded EEG is normal, sleep EEG may provides additional diagnostic information. Falling asleep normally is superior to drug induced sleep as spike activation may occur mainly in the lighter stages of sleep. Sleep deprivation is therefore used to achieve this goal. Occasionally, achieving natural sleep is difficult in young children and drugs need to be used. Benzodiazepines and barbiturates should not be utilized because of their antiepileptic properties and induction of faster EEG frequencies and the drug of choice is chloral hydrate. Chloral hydrate is safe and effective for sleep induction, however, the sleep onset is frequently missed which may alter the EEG interpretation. The sedative effect was not sustained in many children, particularly those with chronic neurological abnormalities. In general, the EEG should be obtained as soon as possible after a seizure as the incidence of epileptiform discharges is highest in the first few days. If the diagnosis is still in question, a repeat EEG is indicated. In one study, an initial EEG was abnormal in 56% of newly diagnosed epilepsy. Repeat EEG identified an additional 11% of those with an initially normal result. Abnormal slowing may occur shortly after the seizure, which can serve to confirm the clinical impression that a seizure has occurred. Up to 20% of children with epilepsy have repeatedly normal EEGs. As well, epileptiform activity may be seen in up to 5% of normal children who may never develop epilepsy, highlighting that epilepsy is a clinical diagnosis.

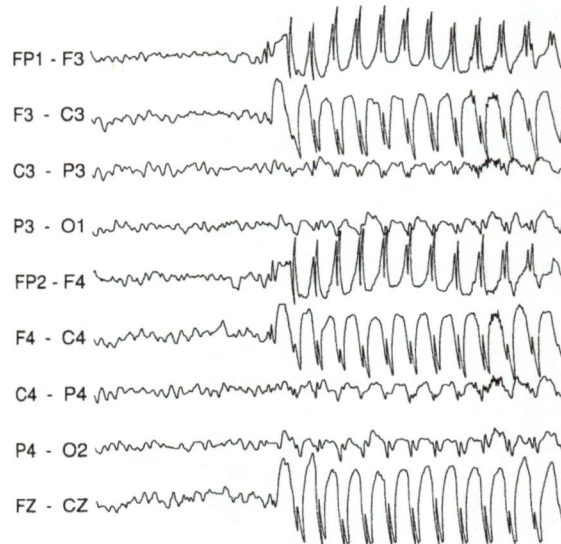

Figure 3: EEG of a child with absence seizures showing the characteristic 3 HZ generalized spike wave discharges.

NEUROIMAGING

Neuroimaging is not routinely recommended for children with benign epilepsy syndromes or primary generalized epilepsy. Computed tomography (CT) scan is satisfactory to screen for large tumors, old infarction, calcifications, and major malformations. CT scan is preferred in emergency situations and for critically ill children who may not tolerate anesthesia. Magnetic resonance imaging (MRI) is superior in identifying cortical developmental lesions (dysplasia), small tumors, malformations, neurocutaneous syndromes, post traumatic and hypoxic insults (Fig. **4**). If both modalities are available, MRI should be performed in preference to CT. Special thin cuts and sequences (coronal flair images) are necessary to assess hippocampal abnormalities if MTS is suspected. MRI is more expensive than CT, not readily available, and requires heavy sedation in young uncooperative children.

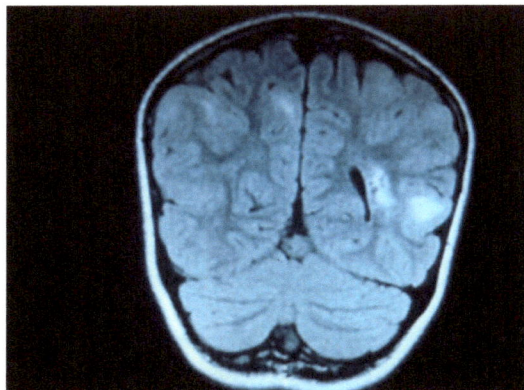

Figure 4: Multiple cortical tubers in a child with tuberous sclerosis and intractable partial epilepsy.

EPILEPSY SYNDROMES

The ILAE classification of epilepsy syndromes (Table **1**) provides valuable genetic, therapeutic, and prognostic information. Syndromes are recognized on the basis of the clinical, developmental, neurological, and EEG characteristics. Some benign syndromes need no treatment (rolandic, occipital epilepsy) while others (juvenile myoclonic epilepsy) may need life long treatment. Overall, the etiology of the syndrome is idiopathic in 25%, cryptogenic in 49%, and symptomatic in 26%. Most children (63%) have localization related (partial) epilepsy syndrome, 12% have a generalized epilepsy syndrome, and 26% are classified as undetermined. Favorable prognosis was associated with idiopathic syndromes, while symptomatic syndromes carry a worse prognosis. Three important syndromes that are frequently missed or misdiagnosed are discussed in the next section. Making the correct diagnosis is critical for proper investigations, management, and counseling.

BENIGN ROLANDIC EPILEPSY

Seizures originating from the centrotemporal (rolandic) region characteristically involve the face and throat with excessive salivation. The seizures are usually simple partial as the child can recall the symptoms of choking, facial twitching, drooling, and inability to speak despite of trying. Seizures mainly occur during sleep and may rapidly generalize. The interictal EEG shows characteristic spike and slow wave discharge in one or both centrotemporal regions that usually activates with sleep. If the history and EEG findings are consistent with this syndrome, imaging studies are not necessary. Rolandic seizures may occur quite infrequently (once in 30%), and therapy often is not recommended, particularly if the seizures are simple partial and the child and family are comfortable without treatment. Indications for treatment include frequent or prolonged seizures and seizures during wakefulness. Controlled release carbamazepine as a single bedtime dose is the drug of choice.

LENNOX-GASTAUT SYNDROME (LGS)

This is a relatively common cryptogenic or symptomatic syndrome of intractable epilepsy due to a wide variety of etiologies. Patients usually present in the first seven years of life with multiple seizure types, particularly nocturnal tonic seizures, but also include atypical absence and atonic seizures. Mental retardation (occasionally progressive) and generalized slow spike-wave discharges (1-2.5 HZ) on EEG are the other two characteristic feature of this syndrome. Fast polyspikes are associated with the tonic seizures. Up to 25% of affected children have history of infantile spasms. Children are usually intractable to multiple AEDs. The best drug combination is valproic acid and lamotrogine.

JUVENILE MYOCLONIC EPILEPSY OF CHILDHOOD

This syndrome occurs in normal young teenagers and is frequently misdiagnosed. Seizures include myoclonic jerks and generalized tonic-clonic seizures upon awakening, and history of absence seizures. Absence seizures at an earlier age (5-10 years) may lead to a diagnosis of absence epilepsy; only a family history of myoclonus or generalized seizures will suggest the diagnosis. The age of onset of myoclonic jerks is 8-15 years and generalized seizures at 9-16 years. The EEG reveals fast (3.5-6 HZ) spike and polyspike wave discharges superimposed on normal background rhythms. In 25%, EEG photic stimulation (repetitively flashing light) results in epileptiform discharges (photoparoxysmal response) and occasionally clinical myoclonus (photoconvulsive response). Some investigators have found a linkage to chromosome 6p. Juvenile myoclonic epilepsy is a chronic disorder and patients may need to be treated for life. Drug options include valproic acid, clobazam, lamotrogine and topiramate. Phenytoin and carbamazepine are contraindicated as they can exacerbate absence and myoclonic seizures.

MANAGEMENT

Once the diagnosis of epilepsy is established, communicating such news to the parents is often difficult and emotional. Most physicians do not feel comfortable dealing with children with neurological disorders such as epilepsy. At the same time, it is important that the transfer of such information is done well as the manner in which neurological bad news is conveyed to parents can significantly influence their emotions, beliefs, and attitudes towards the child and the medical staff. Besides the seizures, children with epilepsy may have behavioral, cognitive, neurological, and sleep disorders. These co-morbidities are the result of the underlying neurological etiology, associated recurring seizures, or antiepileptic drugs (AEDs). Sub-clinical seizures (non-convulsive status epilepticus) can result in cognitive decline and behavioral changes. Some epilepsy syndromes are characterized by cognitive deterioration such as LGS. Parental education and explanations about what to do in acute situation are important as many parents may perform unnecessary maneuvers such as mouth to mouth breathing or inserting objects to keep the mouth open. The parents need to put the child on the side to move the tongue away from the airway and avoid aspiration if the child vomits and remove tight clothing. Certain daily activities need to be modified if the epilepsy is active. Swimming without supervision by a trained adult swimmer, bathing in a full tub, biking without a helmet, and climbing, should be all avoided. Physician should stress the importance of school and discourage overprotection. Some families need psychological counseling to help them deal with epilepsy. Several AEDs are available as shown in Tables **3-6**.

Table 3: List of the available older and newer antiepileptic drugs (AEDs).

Traditional AEDs	New AEDs	Newer AEDs
Phenobarbital (1912)	Clobazam (1991)	Topiramate (1997) Oxcarbazepine (1997)
Phenytoin (1938)	Felbamate (1993)	Tiagabine (1998)
Primidone (1954)	Gabapentin (1994)	Zonisamide (1999) Levetiracetam (2000)
Ethosuximide (1960)	Vigabatrin (1994)	Pregabalin (2004)
Carbamazepine (1974)	Lamotrogine (1995) Fosphyntoin (1996)	
Clonazepam (1975)		
Nitrazepam (1975)		
Valproic Acid (1978)		

Table 4: Comparison between the best five new antiepileptic drugs, ordered according to efficacy, safety, pharmacokinetics, and cost.

Drug	Advantages	Disadvantages
Lamotrogine (Lamictal)	- Broad spectrum - Very effective	- Serious skin rash - Drug interactions - High cost
Topiramate (Topamax)	- Broad spectrum - Very effective - Few drug interactions	- Cognitive side effects - Rare renal stones - High cost
Levetiracetam (Keppra)	- Broad spectrum - Very effective - Few drug interactions	- Behavioral side effects - Rare psychosis - High cost
Gabapentin (Neurontin)	- Very safe - No drug interactions	- Narrow spectrum of action - Short half life - High cost
Vigabatrin (Sabril)	- Very effective - No drug interactions	- Behavioral side effects - High cost - Irreversible retinal toxicity

Table 5: Summary of the older antiepileptic drugs used in children.

Drug	Mechanism	Dose	Interactions	Side Effects
Carbamazepine (Tegretol) 1974	1- Block Na channels 2- Ca channels	20-40 mg/kg divided BID	Decrease the effectiveness of OCP* Increased	Skin rash (10%) ataxia, diplopia, dizziness, nausea, vomiting, blurred vision, pancytopenia, hepatitis, SIADH, irritability,

Table 5: cont….

	Metabolized by the liver to Epoxide (oxidation) 80% protein bound Peak 4-8 hr 1/2 life 5-26 hr Auto-induction	Max 1.6g/d	level if used with pheno-baritone, phenytoin, or valproate (high epoxide) Increased Level if used with erythromycin or cimetidine	personality change, teratogenic (0.5% risk of open neural tube defect), may aggravate myoclonus
Clonazepam (Rivotril) 1975	Chloride channels 80-90% protein bound metabolized by the liver Peak 1hr 1/2 life 18 hr	0.05-0.2 mg/kg divided BID	Rare	Somnolence, irritability, withdrawal seizures, behavioral change, depression, excessive salivation, tolerance
Ethosuximide (Zarontin) 1960	T Ca channels Not protein bound, Metabolized by the liver Peak 3-7 hr 1/2 life 15-68 hr	20-40 mg/kg BID Max 1.5g/d	Decrease the effectiveness of OCP	Abdominal pain, nausea, loss of appetite, vomiting, skin rash, fever, liver dysfunction, pancytopenia, irritability, tiredness in the 1st 1-2 wk, teratogenic
Phenobarbital (Gardinal) 1912	1- Chloride channels 2- Na channels 30% protein bound metabolized by liver (50-80%) and kidney (20-50%) Peak 2-12 hr 1/2 life 82-199 hr	3-6 mg/kg OD Max 200 mg/d	Decrease the effectiveness of OCP, warfarin and theophyllin Increased level with valproate	Skin rash 2% Steven Johnson syndrome, liver induction, sedation, ataxia, impaired coordination irritability, hyper-activity, decreased attention, behavioral change, depression, cognitive deficit,
Phenytoin (Epanutin) 1938	1- Block Na channels 2- Ca channels 90% protein bound Metabolized by the liver Peak 4-8 hr 1/2 life 14-40 hr	4-8 mg/kg divided BID max 400 mg/d	Decrease the effectiveness of OCP Increase free warfarin level Decreased level with alcohol	Hypersensitivity 5% (skin rash, fever, Steven Johnson syndrome, spleenomegaly, hepatitis), vomiting, diplopia, ataxia, dizziness, nystagmus, rickets, hirsutism, gum hyperplasia (10%), chorea
Valproic Acid (Depakene) 1978	1- Na channels 2- T Ca channels 3- Increase brain GABA 90% protein bound Peak 3-8 hr 1/2 life 12-16 hr	20-90 mg/kg divided BID or TID	Asprin (risk of bleeding) Increase phenobarb and free phenytoin level Decrease carbamazepin level (Increase epoxide)	Nausea, vomiting, lethargy, edema, tremor, somnolence, hair loss, unusual alertness, increased appetite, wt gain, thrombocytopeniahepatotoxicity, pancreatitis, teratogenic (2.5% risk of open neural tube defect)

*OCP = Oral contraceptive pills.

Table 6: Summary of the newer antiepileptic drugs used in children.

Drug	Mechanism	Dose	Interactions	Side Effects
Lamotrogine (Lamictal)	1- Na channel 2- Inhibit glutamate and aspartate release 3- GABA inhibitor	5-7 mg/kg divided BID	Decreased level with enzyme inducers Increased level with valproate Inhibit epoxide metabolism	Skin rash 10% (less if started at low dose and increased slowly), Steven Johnson syndrome (higher with valproate), nausea, dizziness, ataxia, headache, insomnia vomiting, diplopia, somnolence, blurred vision,
Topiramate (Topamax)	Saccharide 1-Na channels	5-10 mg/kg divided	Decreased level with enzyme inducers, *e.g.* phenytoin and tegritol	Psychosis, depression sedation, weight loss, dizziness, nephrolithiasis (1.5%), teratogenic, impaired concentration, finger tingling, ataxia,

Table 6: cont….

	2-GABA 3-AMPA effect 4-CA inhibitor	BID		aphasia
Gabapentin (Neurontin)	Competitive inhibitor of amino acid transport into the CNS	25-45 mg/kg divided BID or TID	% absorbed decrease with higher dose (saturable L-AA gut transport)	Ataxia, somnolence, lethargy, dizziness, fatigue, nystagmus, nausea, weight gain, precipitation of myoclonus
Vigabatrin (Sabril)	GABA transaminase inhibitor	50-150 mg/kg divided BID	25% decrease in phenytoin level	Retinal toxicity, irritability, agitation, insomnia, ataxia, drowsiness, confusion, headache, psychosis (2-5%), depression, hallucinations, weight gain, leukopenia

MANAGEMENT

A neurologically normal child with an idiopathic seizure has a 24% recurrence risk in the next year. The risk increases to 37% with prior neurological insult such as cerebral palsy, and 70% if the child had two seizures. It is generally accepted to initiate AED treatment after having 2 seizures within a 6 month period. An abnormal EEG is also a valuable predictor of recurrence. An initial presentation in status epilepticus also increases the risk of recurrence. Children with absence seizures, drop attacks, and infantile spasms are always treated since they usually present with frequent seizures. The choice of AED is dependent upon the type of seizure, syndrome, and EEG patterns. The AED should be effective with few side effects, and cost-effective. Drug options in a decreasing order for partial seizures (with or without secondary generalization) include carbamazepine, phenytoin, phenobarbitone, lamotrigine, valproic acid, topiramate, benzodiazepines, vigabatrin, and gabapentin. Both phenytoin and phenobarbitone are used less often because of their chronic side effects; however, they are very useful in emergency situations. Options for primary generalized seizures include valproic acid, benzodiazepines, phenytoin, phenobarbitone, lamotrigine, topiramate and less commonly carbamazepine. Infantile spasms respond well to steroids, but other choices include vigabatrin, benzodiazepines, valproic acid, lamotrigine, topiramate. Vigabatrin is used less frequently because of the high incidence of visual field restrictions due to irreversible retinal toxicity. Carbamazepine, phenytoin, phenobarbitone, and gabapentin should not be used in infantile spasms or myoclonic seizures. Interestingly, vigabatrin may exacerbate myoclonic seizures despite being effective in children with infantile spasms. Absence epilepsy responds to ethosuximide, valproic acid, lamotrigine, topiramate, and clobazam. Ethosuximide is not effective for any other seizure type. Valproic acid is a better option for children with juvenile absence epilepsy that may be associated with other seizure types. Vigabatrin, carbamazepine, phenytoin, phenobarbitone, and gabapentin should not be used for absence seizures. Atonic seizures (drop attacks) may respond to valproic acid, lamotrigine, topiramate, benzodiazepines, and occasionally phenobarbitone. Both carbamazepine and phenytoin may exacerbate this seizure type.

Most AEDs should be started at a low dose and increased slowly for better tolerance. If the dose is increased with no response, drug levels are indicated to confirm compliance. Other indications for drug levels include drug interactions and toxicity. Routine levels should be discouraged. The best time for obtaining the test is before the morning dose. Monotherapy is best to avoid interactions and side effects and for better compliance. A second AED is added when seizures are resistant to the initial drug, however, this should not be initiated unless a maximum dose is reached with therapeutic levels. Before switching to another drug, the diagnosis should be reevaluated to exclude non-epileptic events and confirm the seizure semiology. For example, staring spells due to absence epilepsy will get worse on carbamazepine. Combination therapy may be necessary for children with multiple seizure types or refractory epilepsy. Synergistic interaction, lamotrigine and valproic acid as an example, results in improved seizure control. However, the incidence of idiosyncratic skin rash is higher with this combination. Therefore the dose of lamotrigine should be started and increased slowly to a maximum of 5 mg/kg/day. Carbamazepine and lamotrigine or topiramate are powerful combination for intractable partial epilepsy, while valproate and topiramate or lamotrogine are favored for intractable generalized seizures. Certain combinations, such as phenobarbital and benzodiazepines should be avoided because of additive CNS depression and effects on muscle tone. Drugs with similar pharmacological actions should not be combined such as phenytoin and carbamazepine. Only under extreme circumstances should more than 2 drugs be used simultaneously to avoid interactions, side effects, and increased cost.

Routine laboratory testing including complete blood count, liver or renal function, is not recommended. Many side effects are idiosyncratic, including skin rash, Stevens-Johnson syndrome, hepatotoxicity, and pancreatitis, cannot be predicted by routine blood tests, unless the child is symptomatic. Valproic acid can be associated with elevations of liver enzymes and serum ammonia. Most cases of fatal hepatotoxicity have been in infants with severe epilepsy. Possibly, many of these children have undiagnosed neurodegenerative or metabolic disorder such as mitochondrial disorders (Alpers Syndrome), which are exacerbated by the valproic acid. Valproic acid should be avoided if progressive or metabolic disorders are suspected. In teenage girls, 5 mg of folic acid should be supplemented daily to prevent open neural tube defects associated with valproic acid. AEDs should be withdrawn after 1-2 years without seizures regardless of the etiology. The recurrence risk is approximately 30-40%. Several studies with 6-12 months treatment have shown only slightly higher recurrence rates. Motor, cognitive, or EEG abnormalities increases the likelihood of future recurrence. However, a normal EEG is not a must before tapering AEDs; it simply increases the recurrence risk, particularly in generalized epilepsy. Drugs are usually tapered over a 6-8 week periods. Longer periods of weaning are not necessary except with phenobarbitone or benzodiazepines to minimize the likelihood of developing withdrawal seizures.

STATUS EPILEPTICUS

Status Epilepticus (SE) is defined as a seizure or series of seizures which continue for at least 30 minutes without return of consciousness between the seizures. SE could be the initial presentation of an epileptic disorder (12%) and 20% of epileptics have SE in the first five years following the diagnosis. Overall, SE is the most common medical neurological emergency in childhood with an incidence of 4-6/10 000 population. It is commoner in younger children, particularly infants with a mortality rate of up to 20%. SE can be classified as idiopathic (35%) or symptomatic (65%) secondary to trauma, neoplasm, stroke, CNS infection or anomalies. Etiologically, it can be secondary to an acute causes (toxic-metabolic) or chronic causes such as established epilepsy (breakthrough or drug related seizures). The chronic group tends to respond more favorably to treatment and have a lower mortality. SE can also be classified as non-convulsive (absence or complex partial) or convulsive. Convulsive SE can be partial motor (epilepsia partialis continua) or generalized (tonic clonic or myoclonic). Non-convulsive SE is characterized by confusion, somnolence, automatic behavior, psychic or cognitive disturbances without any obvious motor phenomena, usually occurring in children with severe epilepsy such as LGS. The management of SE is outlined in Table **7**.

Table 7: Management of pediatric status epilepticus.

Initial Assessment
ABC, Vital signs
Cardiac monitor, Pulse Oximetry, 100% O2
IV access, urgent glucose, gas, and electrolytes
Start anticonvulsant therapy
Focused history and exam (epilepsy, illnesses, trauma, meningitis, focal signs)
Initial Drug treatment
1- Lorazepam 0. 1 mg/kg Buccal or IV (2 mg/min) up to 4 mg/dose <u>OR</u>
Diazepam 0.3 mg/kg IV or 0.4 mg/kg PR (up to 10 mg/dose)
2- Phenytoin 15-20 mg/kg (infuse at <50 mg/min) <u>OR</u>
Fosphenytoin 20 mg/kg IV (<150 mg/min)

Table 7: cont....

Further Steps If No Response
1- Prepare for intubation and ventilation
2- Repeat Lorazepam (8 mg maximum total dose) <u>OR</u>
Repeat Diazepam (20 mg maximum total dose)
3- Phenobarbital 20 mg/kg IV (infuse at <75 mg/min)
4- Additional Phenytoin then Phenobarbital at 10 mg/kg

Refractory Status Epilepticus
1- Team approach including neurology and intensive care unit
2- Consider EEG monitoring, central line, and blood pressure support
3- Additional drug options include:
a- Paraldehyde 0.1 ml/kg PR or IV
b- Midazolam 0.2 mg/kg IV slowly then infuse at 0.75-10 µg/kg/min
c- Propofol 1-2 mg/kg IV then infuse at 2-10 mg/kg/hr
d- Pentobarbital 5-15 mg/kg over 1 hr followed by 0.5-3 mg/kg/hr
e- Thiopental 3-4 mg/kg followed by 0.2 mg/kg/min

Taking a focused history and performing a focused examination are critical to identify medical illnesses, trauma, infection, intoxication, or child abuse. Benzodiazepines are effective (80%) and fast (2. 5 min) in aborting the seizures (Table 7). Lorazepam has longer duration of effect (12-24 hr) when compared to diazepam (15-30 min). Phenytoin is preferred to phenobarbitone to avoid additional respiratory depression, hypotension, or further impairment of consciousness. Fosphenytoin is a phosphate ester prodrug of phenytoin with no propylene glycol leading to fewer side effects (hypotension, arrhythmia, and thrombophlebitis). The physician should be prepared for intubation once phenobarbital is given after benzodiazepines because of additive depressant effects. Other drug options for intractable SE are outlined in Table 7. SE of longer duration tends to be less responsive to drug therapy. Midazolam and Propofol induce anesthesia with rapid clearance and less pronounced hypotensive effects. If used, they should be maintained for 12-24 hr then withdrawn gradually. Pentobarbital is an active metabolite of thiopental, both with possible neuroprotective effects. However, severe hypotention require inatropic therapy. They also have saturable metabolism with accumulation in lipoid tissues resulting in delays in postinfusion recovery. Therefore, midazolam and propofol are increasingly popular when compared to these long acting barbiturates.

INTRACTABLE EPILEPSY

Intractable epilepsy is defined as recurrent seizures that failed to respond to at least three antiepileptic drug trials singly or in combination despite of using maximum doses or doses resulting in therapeutic drug levels. Intractability has been associated with cognitive and behavioral problems and impaired psychosocial development. These children have a high potential for long-term disability and difficulties in adjusting to school. Recurrent seizures also increase the risk of injury and even death. Three treatment modalities are available for such children including the ketogenic diet, epilepsy surgery, and vagal nerve stimulation (VNS). The ketogenic diet consists of three to four parts fat to one part carbohydrate. The nutritional content of all meals must be calculated and each food item weighed. The high fat content and relative absence of carbohydrate produces a persistent ketosis, which appears to have a direct anticonvulsant effect. The level of ketosis can be monitored daily in the urine. The diet is not curative, but it decreases seizure frequency in up to 60% of children. It is also associated with improved awareness, however, it is unpalatable, results in many social limitations, and can be associated with diarrhea, growth failure, stones, and acidosis. The long-term effects on lipid homeostasis needs further study. The diet should be supervised by a well-trained dietitian and continued for 1-2 years. Surgical approaches include focal resection, corpus callosotomy, hemispherectomy, and multiple subpial transections. The procedure selected depends upon the type and localization of the seizures. Children with focal epileptic zone, particularly if a lesion is present on imaging studies, do very well with regional resection. The most commonly performed procedure is temporal lobectomy, which can offer >80% chance of cure. The results of extratemporal resection are similar to those of temporal lobectomy if a lesion is present. Results of non-lesional cases are less successful with <40% success rate. Children with hemispheric syndromes such as hemimegalencephaly or Rasmussen syndrome may have an excellent response to undercutting of the cortex of an entire hemisphere (functional hemispherectomy). Other surgical options include corpus callosotomy for generalized atonic or tonic seizures and multiple subpial transactions for epilepsy involving the primary motor or sensory cortex. The vagus nerve stimulator is surgically implanted under the skin of the lateral chest wall and connected to stimulating electrodes attached to the left vagal nerve. The patient or parents also can activate the stimulator, when a seizure is anticipated, by passing a special magnet over the VNS. VNS is approved as an adjunct treatment for intractable partial epilepsy and LGS. The exact mechanism of action is not known, however, it results in significant seizure reduction in up to 30% of children. The procedure is expensive and requires meticulous follow up.

SUMMARY

This chapter summarized many important aspects of pediatric epilepsy. Seizures in children have wider variations in clinical expression with age specific presentation. Epilepsy syndromes are also more common in children and proper diagnosis provides valuable genetic, therapeutic, and prognostic information. Careful and detailed history remains the cornerstone of an accurate diagnosis. Monotherapy is the best management approach for better compliance and to prevent interactions or side effects. Drug levels and periodic blood investigations are not recommended routinely. If the seizures are intractable to multiple AEDs, the physician could consider ketogenic diet, epilepsy surgery, and vagal nerve stimulation. AEDs should be withdrawn after 1-2 year seizure free interval. Drugs are usually tapered over a 6-8 week periods. Motor, cognitive, and EEG abnormalities increases the likelihood of future recurrence, however, a normal EEG is not a must before tapering AEDs.

BIBLIOGRAPHY

Jan MM: Assessment of the Utility of Pediatric Electroencephalography. Seizure 2002;11(2):99-103.

Jan MM: The Value of Postictal Electroencephalogram In Temporal Lobe Seizures. Ann Saudi Med 1999;19(6):550-553.

Jan MM, Shaabat AO: Clobazam For The Treatment of Intractable Childhood Epilepsy. Saudi Med J 2000;21(7):622-624.

Jan MM, Aquino MF: The Use of Chloral Hydrate In Pediatric Electroencephalography. Neurosciences 2001;6(2):99-102.

Jan MM, Sadler M, Rahey SR: Lateralized Postictal EEG Delta Predicts The Side of Seizure Surgery in Temporal Lobe Epilepsy. Epilepsia 2001;42:402-5.

Jan MM, Neville BGR, Cox TC, Scott RC: Convulsive Status Epilepticus in Children with Intractable Epilepsy is Frequently Focal in Origin. Can J Neurol Sci 2002;29:65-67.

Jan MM, Baeesa SS, Shivji Z: Topiramate For The Treatment of Infants with Early Myoclonic Encephalopathy. Neurosciences 2003;8(2):110-112.

Hassan A, Jan MM, Shaabat AO: Topiramate for The Treatment of Intractable Childhood Epilepsy. Neurosciences 2003;8(4):233-236.

Elsayed AM, Jan MM. Levetiracetam in Intractable Childhood Onset Epilepsy. J Pediatr Neurol 2006;4:97-101.

Jan MM: Intractable Childhood Epilepsy and Maternal Fatigue. Can J Neurol Sci 2006;33(3):306-310.

Jan MM. Potentially Serious Lamotrigine-Related Skin Rash. Neurosciences 2007;12:17-20.

Jan MM, Zuberi SA, Alsaihati BA: Pregabalin: Preliminary Experience in Intractable childhood epilepsy. Ped Neurol 2009;40(5):347-50.

Jan MM. Shuddering attacks are not related to essential tremor. J Child Neurol 2010;25(7):881-3.

Shivji ZM, Al-Zahrani IS, Al-Said YA, Jan MM: Subacute Sclerosing Panencephalitis Presenting with Unilateral Periodic Myoclonic Jerks. Can J Neurol Sci 2003;30(4):384-7.

Jan MM: Clinical Review of Pediatric Epilepsy. Neurosciences 2005;10(4):255-64.

Bahassan NA, Jan MM: Ketogenic diet: Update and Application. Neurosciences 2006;11(4):235-240.

Jan MM, Sadler M, Rahey SR. Electroencephalographic features of temporal lobe epilepsy. Can J Neurol Sci 2010;37: 439-48.

Jan MM: Benign Myoclonic Epilepsy of Infancy: May Not Be So Benign At Diagnosis. Neurosciences 1999;4(4):315.

Jan MM: Folic Acid and Seizures. Eur J Neurol 1999;6(5):619.

CHAPTER 10

Seizure Semiology

Abstract: The diagnosis of epilepsy depends upon a number of factors, particularly detailed and accurate seizure history, or semiology. Other diagnostic data, consisting of electroencephalography (EEG), video-monitoring of the seizures, and magnetic resonance imaging (MRI), are important in any comprehensive epilepsy program, particularly with respect to lateralizing and localizing the seizure focus, if such a focus exists, and with respect to determining the type of seizure or seizure syndrome. The aim of this chapter is to present a survey of important semiologic characteristics of various seizures that provide the historian with observations, which help to lateralize and localize epileptic zones. Clinical semiology is the starting point of understanding a seizure disorder and making the diagnosis of epilepsy. While it may not provide unequivocal evidence of localization of the epileptic focus, nevertheless it usually directs subsequent investigations, whose concordance is necessary for the ultimate localization.

Keywords: Seizure, Epilepsy, Preictal, Ictus, Postictal, Aura, Occipital, Semiology, Conciousness, Awareness, Frontal, Temporal, Parietal.

BACKGROUND

The diagnosis of epilepsy is dependent upon a very detailed and accurate history. The recording of this chronological sequence of recurrent, transient, self-limited, involuntary, alteration in the neurological state, *e.g.* the semiology, must be meticulously sought. It is the quality of this inquiry that allows one to understand the patient's complaints and to provide the diagnosis of epilepsy. Epilepsy is a clinical diagnosis and there is really no other single investigation that can accurately exclude or diagnose epilepsy. The clinical information not only makes the diagnosis, but it also allows the seizures to be classified. An accurate semiologic history is not only important in the diagnosis, but it is most important in determining the region of the brain from which the seizures are arising in patients with intractable epilepsy who are being considered for surgical management. Certainly one would not minimize the importance of electroencephalography (EEG), video-monitoring, and magnetic resonance imaging (MRI) in localization of seizure foci, but discordance of the localization of the clinical semiology with these other tests within the investigative armamentarium raises suspicion about the accuracy of the localization.

SEIZURE HISTORY

As already emphasized, there is no substitution for a carefully obtained history when one initially encounters a patient with epilepsy. Meticulousness is often required in seeking a satisfactorily accurate semiology has many rewards. It provides one of the lost aspects of the Art of Medicine in today's healthcare environment, but in addition to serving the patient it rewards the young epileptologist and sets what hopefully will be a life-long discipline in history taking, and lastly it provides the necessary information to make a diagnosis and to classify the epileptic condition. A previous diagnosis of epilepsy should not necessarily be accepted without a confirmatory history, if there are any reasons to question its quality. Clinical experience is replete with examples in which inaccurate initial histories are accepted and transferred from one document to another, until the suspicious historian realizes that there is discordance in the subsequent investigation, course, diagnosis, and/or management of the patient's seizure disorder. Unfortunately this occurs far too often in residency training programs where the rigid discipline of high quality history taking has been allowed to be compromised. The first encounter often requires: 1) follow-up visits with the patient, *per se*, who may be able to obtain additional information from individuals who have witnessed her/his seizures, 2) phone calls to other witnesses, such as a family member or a friend, 3) formal consultations with such witnesses, or 4) the request of home video taping of seizures when this is possible. The combination of one or all of these strategies should allow the attentive examiner to make as accurate a diagnosis as possible clinically. In the case of very young patients the physician should not slip into the practice of not fully including the patient in the conversation, as the child can often provide valuable additional information, which otherwise might not be realized. In all the strategies, the request for the interviewees to mimic the patients' seizures may actually be the most important information leading to the diagnosis, lateralization and localization! The time of the day when seizures might occur is important as some occur predominantly in sleep (benign Rolandic seizures, tonic seizures in Lennox Gastaut syndrome, and frontal lobe seizures). In order to optimize the quality of the information gained during history taking it is worth remembering that each event may potentially have four stages: preictal, ictal onset (aura), ictus, and postictal as shown in Table **1**.

1- Pre-ictal Phase: The premonitory phase includes the so-called provoking or precipitating factors such as fever, illness, high altitude, lack of sleep, lack of compliance, menstruation, and head injury. However, this stage may also include symptoms that may be somewhat controversial and defy placement in the ictal onset phase. The controversy is usually associated with the event lasting an inordinate length of time, *e.g.* tens of minutes, hours or even, in some cases, days. These are referred to prodromal symptoms and should not be confused with seizure onset. Such events are not common, but should not be rejected out of hand, as very occasionally they may form part of the true seizure semiology, in which case they may have localizing value with respect to seizure onset (see below). Some examples of such include headaches, behavioural irritability, and personality change.

Table 1: Seizure history taking and its significance.

FEATURES	SIGNIFICANCE
1- Before seizure onset	
Prodrome	May precedes generalized tonic clonic seizures
Environment of occurrence	To exclude syncope or pseudoseizures
Time of the day (*e.g.* upon awakening)	Myoclonic or primary generalized epilepsy
Precipitants or triggers	Reflex or photosensitive epilepsy
Association with sleep	Rolandic or frontal lobe epilepsy
2- At seizure onset	
Aura	Lobe of origin (*e.g.* occipital if visual)
Focal onset	Lateralization and/or localization
3- During the seizure	
Progression	Identify the involved brain regions
Aphasia	Dominant hemisphere
Awareness & consciousness	Simple versus complex partial or generalized
Duration	Status epilepticus
4- After the seizure (postictal)	
Confusion/amnesia	Suggests complex partial or generalized
Unilateral headache	Ipsilateral seizure origin
Weakness (Todd's paresis)	Contralateral hemispheric origin
Visual field defect	Occipital lobe involvement
Dysphasia	Dominant hemispheric involvement

2- Ictal Onset: Because of the dramatic aspects of a generalized tonic-clonic seizure, which often is thought, at least transiently, to be an agonal event by many lay people, there is a tendency to consider this as the "seizure" in totality, with no significance attached to a possible importance of the preceding or post-ictal symptomatology. However, as already indicated and as well known, the very first event in the chronological sequence of events in a seizure is the most important feature for the localization of a seizure focus, in the case of partial seizures. The history of any brief focal signs or symptoms (aura) at the beginning of the more dramatic seizure must be obtained. When a history is considered to be of poor quality the most common criticism is the failure to obtain a satisfactory determination of this very first event in the semiology, when in fact there is such an event. The patient usually refers to this part of the seizure as the "warning". The historian needs to be perfectly satisfactorily convinced that indeed the initial event has been elucidated. This requires good listening ability and intelligent questioning by the clinician. This importance can be appreciated in an example of a semiology that consists of an abnormal hallucinatory taste, followed by a rising epigastric sensation, followed by deviation of the head and eyes, and then clonic movements of the thumb. Each of these alone may lead to the conclusion that the seizure focus is in a different location. For example, if the clonic movements of the thumb are interpreted as the initial event then the contralateral dorsolateral motor neocortex would be the suggested focus, as opposed to the contralateral premotor cortex (head and eye deviation), the inferomesial temporal lobe (rising epigastric sensation), or the contralateral supraSylvian inferior Rolandic cortex (abnormal taste). In the foregoing example of the simple partial seizure onset with four different components the latter three events are not without importance, as they are interpreted as reflecting the spread of the seizure discharge. Such spread of the seizure over the cortex has the potential of detracting somewhat from the certainty of the clinical localization. As outlined in the foregoing paragraph the four components noted in the example of the seizure semiology can be attributed to relatively specific cortical areal representations. Such cortical areas, which are associated with clinically recognizable function, have come to be known as so-called "functional", or "eloquent", cortex, in contrast to those areas of cortex, which have no such clearly recognizable function; the latter have been labeled by some as "silent", or "non-eloquent", cortex. The neurophysiological student will immediately recognize the arbitrary and somewhat naïve nature of such an assumption, especially if that assumption carries the implication that this is indeed physiologically functionless cortex. However, putting that aside this differentiation does have clinical use, so long as one remembers that a seizure focus may begin in this so-called silent cortex with the first clinical event being recognized when the spread of the seizure impinges upon an area of clinically "functional" cortex. Thus, while in theory one might consider this as an example of false localization, nevertheless the clinical usefulness of localization of epileptic foci from semiology derives from the fact that while perhaps an area of silent cortex is the focus, nevertheless this is usually in the immediate vicinity of the nearby involved "functional" cortex, which has led to the clinical localization.

3- Ictal Phase: The ictus is usually associated with an alteration in consciousness. This alteration may be a loss of consciousness, as in primary generalized tonic-clonic seizures or simply an "altered" state, which is characteristically seen in complex partial seizures of temporal lobe origin. The alterations in the latter may be such that the naïve observer may interpret the patient's state as one of full consciousness, particularly when associated automatic behavior (automatisms) appears normal, or near normal (see below). Staring due to complex partial seizures should not be confused with that of absence seizures. Hyperventilation for 3 minutes can induce an absence seizure and results in quick diagnosis during the clinic visit. Additional helpful differentiating features are summarized in Table **2**. There are times when referral notes will refer to two or three different seizure types. It is very important to sort this out, as more than one seizure type suggests more than one seizure focus. Bitemporal seizures may occur for reasons which are not the subject of this paper, but other instances of more than one epileptic focus in a given patient is a very, very uncommon eventuality. Usually in these instances the two or three seizure types are simply extensions of single seizure semiology. Perhaps the commonest such example is a typical complex partial seizure with simple partial onset and secondary generalization, in which an interpretation is that these three components of a single seizure semiology represent three separate seizure types, as opposed to simply an extension of the same seizure focus.

Table 2: Differentiating staring due to absence from that of complex partial seizures.

FEATURES	ABSENCE	COMPLEX PARTIAL
Sleep activation	None	Common
Hyperventilation	Induces the seizures	No activating effect
Seizure frequency	Frequent (daily)	Less frequent
Seizure onset	Abrupt	Slow
Aura	None	If preceded by a simple partial seizure
Automatism	Rare	Common
Progression	Minimal	Evolution of features
Cyanosis	None	Common

Table 2: cont....

Motor signs	Rare, or minimal	Common
Seizure duration	Brief (usually <30 sec)	Minutes
Postictal confusion or sleep	None	Common
Postictal dysphasia	None	Common in seizures originating from the dominant hemisphere

4- Post-ictal Phase: The post-ictal period may also have clinically valid localizing factors, even though they may be seen in this phase at the end of the seizure. These post-ictal changes take the form of deficits of function. In a primary generalized seizure, for example, there may be a post-ictal deficit with localizing value. For example, post-ictal weakness (Todd's paresis) or visual deficits will point to involvement of the associated functional cortex in the contralateral hemisphere. Post-ictal dysphasia will suggest involvement of the dominant hemisphere. It is not uncommon to see a patient whose referral notes have clearly stated the diagnosis of primary generalized seizures, only to find out upon close questioning of those witnessing the post-ictal periods of the patient's seizures valuable information of localizing and/or lateralizing value in the diagnosis of partial seizures. Severe post-ictal headache is most common following occipital lobe or generalized tonic-clonic seizures.

CLINICAL SEMIOLOGY

While the quality of the determination of the semiology, as derived from the history, may be superseded by semiological features identified by good quality video- monitoring, yet the clinical semiology, along with EEG evaluation, medical imaging (MRI) and neuropsychological assessment are all important in identifying the epileptic focus in patients with intractable epilepsy who are being considered for possible epilepsy surgery. It is the concordance of these assessments, which is usually necessary for the recommendation of epilepsy surgery; it has similar importance in the prognosis of such surgery. In discussing semiology it is helpful to consider some common categories of semiologic features, especially when differentiating frontal lobe (FL) from temporal lobe (TL) seizures – the two regions most frequently affected by partial epilepsy and the most common difficult differentiation of partial seizures. Using the features outlined in Table **3**, seizures have been reported to be reasonably accurately localizable to the frontal or temporal lobes in the majority of patients. Other important lateralizing and localizing semiologic features of partial and secondarily generalized seizures are summarized in Table **4**. They can be grouped into one of the following four categories, 1) automatism, 2) speech, 3) motor, and 4) autonomic features.

Table 3: Semiology of frontal versus temporal lobe seizures.

FEATURES	FRONTAL LOBE	TEMPORAL LOBE
Seizure frequency	Frequent, often daily	Less frequent
Sleep activation	Characteristic	Less common
Seizure onset	Abrupt, explosive	Slower
Progression	Rapid	Slower
Initial motionless staring	Less common	Common
Automatisms	Less common	More common and longer
Bipedal automatism	Characteristic	Rare
Complex postures	Early, frequent, and prominent	Late, less frequent and less prominent
Hyperkinetic signs	Common	Rare
Somatosensory symptoms	Common	Rare
Speech	Loud vocalization (screaming, moaning)	Verbalization speech in non-dominant seizures
Seizure duration	Brief	Longer

Table 3: cont....

Secondary generalization	Common	Less common
Postictal confusion	Less prominent, short	More prominent, longer
Postictal dysphasia	Rare, unless it spreads to the dominant temporal lobe	Common in dominant temporal lobe seizures

Table 4: Important semiologic features and their lateralizing and/or localizing value.

Semiologic features	Lateralization and/or localization
1- Automatism	
Oral automatism Unilateral limb automatism	Temporal lobe, typically hippocampal
Unilateral eye blinks	Ipsilateral to seizure origin
Bipedal automatisms	Ipsilateral to seizure origin
Ictal spitting or drinking	Frontal lobe seizures
Ictal laughter (Gelastic)	Right temporal seizures
Postictal nose wiping Postictal cough	Hypothalamic, mesial temporal or frontal cingulate origin
	Ipsilateral temporal lobe seizures
	Temporal lobe seizures
2- Language abnormalities	
Ictal speech arrest	Temporal lobe seizures, usually dominant hemisphere
Ictal speech preservation	Temporal lobe seizures, usually non-dominant hemisphere
Postictal dysphasia	Dominant hemisphere involvement
3- Motor abnormalities	
Early nonforced head turn Late forced head turn	Ipsilateral to seizure origin
Eye deviation	Contralateral to seizure origin
Focal clonic jerking	Contralateral to seizure origin
Asymmetric clonic ending Dystonic limb posturing	Contralateral to seizure origin, peri-rolandic
	Ipsilateral to seizure origin
Tonic limb posturing	Contralateral to seizure origin
Fencing posture	Contralateral to seizure origin
Figure of 4 sign	Contralateral frontal lobe (supplementary motor) seizures
Unilateral ictal paresis	Contralateral to the extended limb, usually temporal lobe
Postictal Todd's paresis	Contralateral to seizure origin
	Contralateral to seizure origin
4- Autonomic features	
Ictus emeticus	Right temporal seizures
Ictal urinary urge	Right temporal seizures
Piloerection (goose bumps)	Left temporal seizures

1- Automatism: Automatisms are repetitive involuntary, purposeless or semi-purposeful movements that are usually inappropriate, but indeed occasionally may simulate relatively normal movements. The latter are usually recognized as being abnormal by their inappropriateness under the circumstances at the time. Oro-alimentary automatisms, consisting of lip smacking, sucking, swallowing, and/or chewing movements, especially occurring near the beginning of a seizure, are suggestive of temporal lobe epilepsy (TLE), originating in the limbic (inferomesial) portion of the lobe. While these automatisms have localizing value, yet they have no lateralizing value. Unilateral eye blinking (winks) is a rare phenomenon that is reported to have ipsilateral localizing value onset. It should not be confused with hemi-facial rhythmical repetitive clonic jerking associated with contralateral motor cortex onset.

2- Language Abnormalities: Speech disturbances during seizures include receptive, expressive, or global dysphasia. The lateralizing value of ictal speech preservation or arrest is described in Table **4**. Ictal verbalization, consisting of understandable names, verbal phrases or sentences should be distinguished from guttural vocalizations such as moaning, grunting, and/or screaming. While vocalizations have no specific lateralizing value, nevertheless they appear to be more commonly seen in frontal lobe seizures.

Naming defects (dysnomia) and paraphasic errors are easily demonstrable during seizures. Postictal dysphasia is a very useful lateralizing sign, but it may not be detected unless the monitoring staff routinely specifically tests post-ictal speech function (Table **5**). Post-ictal dysphasia, like onset or ictal dysphasia, points to a focus in the dominant hemisphere. Non-dominant hemisphere seizures can also interfere with speech function. It may be simply on the basis of post-ictal mental confusion. Speech arrest may occur at the onset of a seizure from involvement of the speech areas, but can also occur from involvement of the inferior Rolandic (sensory-motor) cortex and the supplementary motor area.

Table 5: Examination of patients during the seizure for semiologic characteristics.

Examination	Significance
Response to communication	Level of awareness
Speech (naming, reading)	Dominant hemispheric involvement
Memory (presenting words or phrases for later recall)	Temporal lobe involvement
Distractibility	Frontal lobe involvement
Response to passive eye opening	To exclude pseudoseizure (tight closure)
Response to physical stimulation	Attention, motor dysfunction
Weakness or lack of motor control	Contralateral seizure origin
Plantar extensor response	Post-ictal paresis

3- Motor Abnormalities: Motor signs may be positive, involving involuntary clonic and/or tonic movements, abnormal posturing, dystonia, and head and/or eye deviation. Negative motor signs include muscle weakness or paralysis. Positive motor signs should be distinguished from automatisms, which were described earlier. Whereas in the latter there are usually some fragments, albeit perhaps very brief, which could be construed as semi purposeful or purposeful movements, none such movements occur in the case of clonic and tonic movements. When abnormal bilateral motor activity occurs, a careful examination of the time of onset on each side and the symmetry of the movement between the sides is warranted. Early occurrence or more vigorous activity on one side suggests a contralateral focus, *e.g.* similar to the presence of a post-ictal hemiparesis. While early asymmetric motor activity usually correlates with the seizure origin, late asymmetry may suggest seizure propagation. Head deviation at the onset of a seizure in the presence of normal consciousness is a strong indication of a contralateral mid frontal dorsolateral cortical focus. Non-forced head rotation – a voluntary-like head turn – when it appears early is reported to be often associated with ipsilateral hand automatisms, and is usually toward the hemisphere of seizure origin. Be aware of the initial head turn that may be no more than a response to an external stimulus in a partially responsive patient. Later head turn is due to seizures arising from the contralateral hemisphere, more commonly accompanying temporal lobe than frontal lobe seizures, occurring in the later stage of the seizures. Eye deviation is usually associated with forced head turning and occurs in the same direction. Striking head and eye deviation can occur with contralateral occipital seizures; these may even be accompanied by turning of the upper body! Post-ictal head deviation is assumed to be passive and thus suggestive of ipsilateral frontal lobe involvement. Focal clonic jerking is one of the indisputable localizing and lateralizing features, with the focus situated in the contralateral motor cortex, with further localization within that cortex from a knowledge of the homunculus, *i.e.* facial twitching from the inferior cortex, hand clonus from the middle dorsolateral motor cortex and clonic leg movements from the medial motor cortex. Such focal clonic activity may be seen late in temporal lobe seizures, assumed to be the result of spread of the epileptic discharge out of the temporal lobe. "Asymmetric ending of clonus" refers to unilateral clonic jerking occurring in a terminal phase of generalized seizures, interpreted as the final clonus occurring ipsilateral to the seizure onset, as a result of spread to, and termination in, the contralateral hemisphere. In contrast to the localizing significance of clonic motor activity, tonic movements do not have predictable specificity of localization and lateralization. Sustained unilateral dystonic posturing of the arm and leg has been attributed to spread to the contralateral basal ganglia. Typical hand posture involves wrist flexion, finger flexion at the metacarpo-phalangeal joints, finger extension at the inter-phalangeal joints, and thumb adduction. Unilateral tonic limb posturing is suggestive of contralateral hemispheric seizure origin.

Asymmetric tonic limb posturing (figure of 4 Sign) is usually observed during the early tonic phase of partial seizures as they become secondarily generalized. One arm is extended at the elbow while the other is flexed at the elbow, giving the appearance of a figure of 4. Both arms are slightly raised in front of the chest. The seizure onset is contralateral to the extended limb, and is usually temporal lobe in origin. Unilateral ictal limb paresis may or may not persist into the postictal phase and is associated with contralateral hemispheric origin. Postictal weakness (Todd's paresis) suggests contralateral hemispheric origin. The weakness may not be obvious to the observer; therefore, power should be specifically tested during and after seizures (Table **5**). Asking the patient to point to the ceiling with each hand would test for weakness, as well as, for the level of awareness by following the command.

4- Autonomic symptomatology: Postictal vomiting has no lateralizing value; however, early ictal vomiting (ictus emesis) may suggest right temporal lobe origin. Ictal vomiting can also be seen in the benign occipital epilepsies. Ictal urinary urge and piloerection (goose bumps) are rare and are usually associated with temporal lobe seizures as shown in Table **4**.

TEMPORAL LOBE SEIZURES

Temporal lobe seizures are the commonest site of origin of partial seizures and account for about two thirds of cases of intractable epilepsy that become managed surgically in our experience. The seizures are typically complex partial, with or without simple partial onset. The semiologic features of TLE, some of which have been noted earlier, are nearly boundless. Jackson described the so-called "dreamy state" in seizure semiology in the 19th century. With the comparison of clinical observations and responses to intraoperative stimulation studies, the Montreal school described these psychic phenomena as interpretative illusions or experiential hallucinations. Oro-alimentary automatisms are common, occurring in approximately 70% of cases of limbic (hippocampal) seizures compared to 10% of patients with extra-limbic seizures. Unilateral dystonic posturing of an arm is classical of contralateral temporal lobe epilepsy. This is often present with other more easily appreciated automatisms in the other arm, *e.g.* repetitive purposeless finger movements. This has led to the appreciation that unilateral upper limb automatisms have localizing value, implicating the ipsilateral TL. Commonly the automatisms appear rather symmetrical initially, the clearly dystonic limb appearing later in the established automatism. However, unilateral automatisms without contralateral dystonia have a lower lateralizing value. Postictal nose rubbing or wiping is an uncommon form of unilateral limb automatism resulting from parasympathetic overactivity. It is usually associated with ipsilateral temporal lobe seizures. Postictal coughing may also be associated with TL seizures. Olfactory auras usually consist of poorly recognizable, always unpleasant, foul smell and historically were attributed to the uncus of the temporal lobe, thus becoming known as "uncal" or "uncinate" fits. More recently it has been realized that this localization may be less specific than originally thought. Fear is another limbic aura, considered to be amygdaloid in origin. For this localization, it must be "primary fear", and not simply the often secondary fear that is experienced by the epileptic patient in response to the realization that "another" seizure is about to occur. Primary fear cannot be reduced, or altered, by the patient. Usually there is an accompanying fearful facial countenance. Patients with left temporal lobe seizures cannot read normally post-ictally. Post-ictal dysphasia is more common in TLE than in frontal lobe foci. The relationship of behavioral aggression and TLE has been the subject of a broad cross section of the literature. These behavioral oddities may also include sexual features, fetishes, and hypergraphia. TL seizures can, and have been, separated by some into the much more common (80%+) limbic, or antero-infero-mesial, and neocortical, TLE, depending upon origins in the amygdala/entorhinal/hippocampal area and neocortex, respectively. The auditory illusory auras may originate from either side temporal neocortex.

FRONTAL LOBE SEIZURES

The seizures of frontal lobe epilepsy (FLE) are usually briefer, are associated with less post-ictal confusion, are more motor in characteristics, are more likely to be involved with secondary generalization, are less likely to demonstrate psychic/emotional/affective phenomena, are more likely to exhibit a rapid onset and offset, and are more likely to occur nocturnally than other partial seizures as shown in Table **3**. Geier and colleagues noted that the automatisms of frontal lobe epilepsy suggested that they were of a "forced nature"; hence, they exhibit some differences from those of other origins. These collectively stand in particular contrast to temporal lobe seizures. While there are no clearly pathognomonic features of FLE, apart from the clearly localizable clonic seizures of the motor cortex, yet some generalizations with respect to the semiology of seizures arising in the frontal lobe may be made regarding their sites of origin. The frontal areas that emerge, representing potentially different are: 1) fronto-polar, 2) orbito-frontal, 3) premotor, including the supplementary motor area (SMA), 4) dominant opercular, and 5) Rolandic. The latter is more logically considered along with its post-central sensory counterpart (somatosensory cortex), under the designation of "Rolandic", or central, seizures. In the other categories of seizures there may be various combinations of the general characteristics of frontal lobe seizures.

1- Fronto-polar: Seizures of fronto-polar origin are often from scars following head injuries. They have the greatest likelihood of simply being characterized by what appear clinically to be primary generalized seizures, *e.g.* generalized tonic-clonic seizures without a simple partial onset. However, as noted in the foregoing, they may have some of the general characteristics of FLE, especially contralateral head deviation.

2- Orbito-frontal: Orbito-frontal seizures may have semiology that mimics temporal lobe seizures in which case the origin is usually attributed to the posterior part of the orbital cortex. Once again, however, it may involve, in various combinations, other frontal lobe semiology, especially contralateral head and eye deviation.

3- Premotor: Head and eye deviation with varying bilateral tonic posturing is the commonest seizure characteristic of premotor seizures. When the deviation occurs at the onset of the seizure when consciousness is intact it has significant localizing value to the contralateral frontal cortex. When it occurs during the seizure in an unconscious patient, it is of little localizing value. Those seizures arising in the mid part of the frontal lobe have a prominent bilateral tonic posturing. Bipedal automatisms may take the form of symmetric bicycling or kicking movements. Prominent leg movements favor involvement of the supplementary motor area. The so-called "fencing posture" is classically associated with the contralateral FL, particularly the SMA. The SMA is really a specialized part of the premotor area, involving the cortex immediately anterior to the precentral sulcus medially and at the upper part of the dorsolateral cortex. It is specialized in that is represents a second motor homunculus. This complex posture is characterized by abduction, external rotation, and partial flexion of the contralateral arm at the shoulder, contralateral deviation of the head and eyes such that they "look at" the contralateral arm, extended ipsilateral arm downwards and backwards, and with the feet apart so as to support the partially contralaterally rotated trunk. Occasionally, the upper limb is also flexed at the elbow with the hand raised to the face that has turned forcefully towards it. There is occasionally guttural, ill-understood speech.

4- Dominant opercular: A seizure origin involving the supraSylvian dominant frontal cortex usually begins with an alteration in speech. The alteration may be typical dysphasic speech, a form of non-specific guttural speech, or an arrest of speech. As noted earlier, it is an important, localizing feature post-ictally when there is dysphasia.

5- Rolandic: The pre- and post-central gyri are considered as a unit, as the majority of Rolandic seizures combine both motor and sensory components, which carry the clear cut features of involvement of the contralateral Rolandic cortex. Sensory features can be positive (*e.g.* pins and needles, pain, pricking, tingling) or negative (numbness). Elementary paraesthesiae are reported to be the most characteristic of seizures arising in the post-central gyrus. Lewin and Phillips described a patient with the simple partial onset of severe pain arising in the contralateral post-central gyrus. In pure sensory seizures there is nearly always dysfunction of the part involved, which may be awkwardness, typical sensory ataxia, or paralysis. In the case of the latter, some have referred to these sensory seizures as "inhibitory seizures" – a very controversial phenomenon. One of the characteristic features of Rolandic seizures is the spread (intracortically) within the Rolandic cortex, *e.g.* sensory and/or motor, over contiguous parts of the associated homunculus. This, therefore, results in consecutive adjacent parts of the body being involved in seizure activity, which clinically is reflected in a "march" from one place on the body to another. Unlike the tonic activity associated with seizures arising outside of the Rolandic cortex, which often has unreliable localizing and lateralizing value, Rolandic motor activity is clonic and is unambiguously localizing to the contralateral motor cortex in the area of the homunculus from which it arises, and usually is associated with transient post-ictal weakness in the involved part.

OCCIPITAL LOBE SEIZURES

A visual aura may be positive, consisting of visual phenomena such as flickering lights, spots, lines, images, or negative in which part of the visual field is defective. Epileptic visual hallucinatory auras should be distinguished from migrainous auras, which develop gradually over 5 minutes and lasts for longer periods of time and with no disruption in the level of consciousness. In this situation, a relatively stereotyped headache usually occurs during or within 60 minutes of the visual aura. Traditionally it has been held that the occipital cortex had the highest threshold with respect to the development of seizures, thus standing in marked contrast to the limbic temporal lobe. Occipital lobe seizures may be heralded by visual auras, *e.g.* illusions or hallucinations, but may begin with auras that are more suggestive of nearby neocortex. When they involve the visual system the involvement will include the contralateral visual (occipital) and/or posterior temporal neocortex. Within this cortex there is a neurophysiological hierarchy, with increasing perceptual sophistication from the cortex of the occipital pole to the posterior temporal cortex. Epileptic discharge in the polar region (Area 17) results in elementary visual features, which lack form, colour, depth, and movement and tend to be fixed in a predictable area of the contralateral visual field. Seizures arising in the more anteriorly situated occipital visual association areas (Areas 18 and 19) exhibit increasing evidence of more elaborate visual hallucinations, with the features of recognizable form, colour, depth, and movement, usually confined to the contralateral half of the visual field. The abnormal epileptic visual abnormalities reach fully developed complex hallucinations from foci in the posterior temporal cortex. These may be illusory, but may represent perfectly normal form with people, environmental structures, landscapes, etc, and involve central vision, occupying the whole of the visual field. Most seizures with these complex visual illusions originate in the non-dominant posterior temporal neocortex.

LIMITATIONS OF CLINICAL SEMIOLOGY

Seizure semiology has some limitations in lateralizing and localizing the seizure origin. Many semiologic features have high positive predictive values; however, each feature has some potential to falsely localize the seizure onset. False localization should be suspected if the onset of clinical seizures occurs earlier than the onset of ictal EEG discharge. The EEG onset should either precede or be simultaneous with the clinical seizure onset. A number of false localizations raise the possibility of multifocal epilepsy. Several seizures have to be recorded to overcome this possibility. Rathke and colleagues showed that seizure semiology localized seizure onset in only 67% of patients with multifocal epilepsy. Another issue that must be remembered is that much of the observational data of seizure semiology has been derived from video-EEG monitored patients with intractable epilepsy. These patients may have semiologic differences when compared to patients with non-intractable epilepsy. As well, some seizures of monitored patients are precipitated by antiepileptic drug withdrawal. In this situation, the seizure duration and intensity, as well as the likelihood of secondary generalization, are increased. In spite of this, however, available evidence indicates that seizure onset characteristics are not substantially altered and therefore appear to be the same as habitual seizures. However, rapid generalization can erase the subjective aura from the patient's memory and can give the objective observe increased difficulty of recognizing the individual components of the seizures. Most of the semiologic features that were summarized in Table **3** are useful for hemispheric lateralization, whereas few features are helpful for seizure localization. For example, dystonic limb posturing is more useful for hemispheric lateralization because of its high predictive value; however, it can be observed in seizures arising from either the frontal or temporal lobes. In contrast, bipedal automatisms, such as bicycling movements, are usually observed with frontal lobe seizures, but it does not suggest the side of seizure onset. Therefore, the localizing value of recorded seizures is greater when it is based on concordance of multiple semiologic features than when based on an isolated feature. Lastly it must be noted that most literature descriptions of seizure semiology have been based on adult patients. Temporal lobe epilepsy is more difficult to recognize in children. Childhood TL seizures are less stereotyped and more likely to exhibit prominent tonic posturing or myoclonic jerks. These motor components become less prominent with increasing age. Likewise, frontal lobe seizures in children appear different from those in adults. Hyper motor activity, complex motor automatisms, and secondary generalizations are rarely encountered in children. In general, some semiologic features of partial seizures in children increased with age, such as automatisms, unresponsiveness, dystonic posturing, and secondary generalization, while other features decreased with age, such as asymmetric clonic movements and symmetric tonic posturing.

SUMMARY

Seizure history and video recordings should be reviewed carefully to detect as many useful semiologic features as possible. It is essential to record multiple seizures in intractable patients to establish the consistency of the semiologic features, particularly if surgery is considered. A representative seizure should also be shown to the patient's parents or relatives to confirm that habitual seizures were captured. Analysis of the development and sequence of multiple semiologic features can identify the seizure initiation and propagation. This information should be correlated with EEG and MRI findings. Seizure origin is identified more accurately if ictal EEG onset is concordant with seizure semiology. Therefore, the clinical implications of recorded seizures should be assessed in parallel with information from the clinical history, video-EEG, and imaging studies. Clinical semiology is the starting point of understanding a seizure disorder and making the diagnosis of epilepsy. While it may not provide unequivocal evidence of localization of the epileptic focus, nevertheless it usually directs subsequent investigations, whose concordance is necessary for the ultimate localization.

BIBLIOGRAPHY

Jan MM, Girvin JP: Seizure Semiology: Value in Identifying Seizure Origin. Can J Neurol Sci 2008;35:22-30.

Jan MM: The Value of Seizure Semiology in Lateralizing and Localizing Partially Originating Seizures. Neurosciences 2007;12(3):185-90.

Jan MM: Clinical Review of Pediatric Epilepsy. Neurosciences 2005;10:255-64.

CHAPTER 11

Febrile Seizures

Abstract: Febrile seizures are the most common seizure disorder in children <5 years of age. They occur in 2-5% of children, but the incidence has been reported as high as 14% in certain populations. This has been attributed to higher rates of consanguinity. However, racial and geographic variations may also be important. Most febrile seizures are brief, do not require any specific treatment or workup, and have benign prognoses. Generalists and pediatricians are frequently faced with anxious parents and are required to make rational decisions regarding the workup and management of these children. Physicians are subsequently required to provide counseling and information about the prognoses to the involved families. The aim of this chapter is to provide an updated overview of febrile seizures and review the most recent diagnostic and therapeutic recommendations.

Keywords: Seizure, Epilepsy, Fever, Typical, Atypical, Meningitis, Encephalitis, EEG, MRI, Dravet syndrome, Febrile plus syndrome.

DEFINITIONS

A febrile seizure is defined as a seizure accompanied by fever without central nervous system infection, occurring in infants and children 6 months to 5 years of age. The majority occurs in children between 12-22 months. It is generally accepted that a febrile seizure is associated with a temperature of at least 38.5° C, no acute systemic metabolic abnormalities that may predispose to seizures, and no history of afebrile seizures. Febrile seizures can be simple (typical) or complex (atypical), based on their clinical characteristics. Simple febrile seizures are the most common (85%) and are characterized by a brief generalized seizure, specifically without any lateralizing features. Complex febrile seizures are focal, prolonged (>15 minutes), and/or multiple within 24 hours of the same febrile illness. Complex febrile seizures are less common accounting for <15% of febrile seizures. An initial simple febrile seizure may be followed by complex seizures, but the majority of children who develop complex febrile seizures do so from the onset. When an initial seizure is prolonged, subsequent recurrences are more likely to be prolonged. Febrile status epilepticus accounts for 5% of febrile seizures and for up to 25% of all status epilepticus in children.

FEBRILE ILLNESS

The majority of children have their febrile seizures on the first day of illness. In some cases the seizure is the first manifestation that the child is ill, *i.e.* before the parents detect the fever. The degree of fever is variable, and approximately 75% have temperatures of 39° C or higher at the time of the seizure. Recurrent febrile seizures do not necessarily occur with the same degree of fever as the first episode and do not occur every time the child has a fever. Although it is often contended that a febrile seizure is more likely to occur when temperature increases rapidly, there is no scientific data to support this belief. Febrile seizures occur more commonly during viral than bacterial infections. Some viral infections, such as roseola (herpes virus 6), appear to be particularly prone to be associated with seizure activity in infants according to Hall and colleagues who observed seizures in up to 13% of such children. In another study, roseola accounted for up to 33% of first febrile seizures and frequently was of the complex type. Interestingly, when gastroenteritis is the cause of the fever, seizures are extremely uncommon, *i.e.* has an inverse relationship.

GENETICS

Genetic factors appear to be important in the expression of febrile seizures and in the relationship to future epilepsy. Males generally have a higher incidence with a male to female ratio of about 1. 5-2:1. Among first-degree relatives of children with febrile seizures, 7-31% had history of febrile seizures. Other siblings of an affected family have a 20-30% risk of having febrile seizures. In addition, monozygotic twins have a much higher concordance rate than dizygotic twins, in whom the rate is similar to that of other siblings.

Susceptibility to febrile seizures has been recently linked to several genetic loci in different families, including the long arm of chromosome 8q13-21, chromosome 19p, chromosome 2q23-24, and chromosome 5q14-15. The suggested mode of inheritance is autosomal dominant. The recently described syndrome of generalized epilepsy with febrile seizures plus has been mapped to chromosome 2q. Involved children have febrile seizures that continue beyond six years of age or associated with afebrile generalized seizures or other seizure types such as absence, myoclonic, or atonic seizures. The epilepsy typically remits by mid-adolescence. A subsequent report described other unrelated families with the same clinical syndrome. Genetic analyses suggested autosomal dominant inheritance with a penetrance of approximately 60%. In one of the families, the syndrome was linked to chromosome 19q and a mutation was identified in the β-subunit of sodium channels. A similar autosomal dominant syndrome was studied in two French families. The gene was mapped to chromosome 2q21-q33 and two mutations of the gene encoding the α-subunit of sodium channels were found. In summary, the evidence in febrile seizures suggests autosomal dominant inheritance, low penetrance, variable expression, and locus heterogeneity.

RECURRENCE OF FEBRILE SEIZURES

Children with febrile seizures are at risk for developing recurrent febrile seizures. A major factor influencing the recurrence rate is the age of the infant at the time of the first seizure. The overall recurrence rate is approximately 30-35% and increases to 50% after the second febrile seizure. However, the values vary with age from as high as 50-65% in infants <1 year of age to as low as 20% in older children. A prospective cohort study of 428 children with a first febrile seizure identified four important factors influencing seizure recurrence; 1) age <1 year, 2) family history of febrile seizures, 3) low grade fever, and 4) seizures following brief fevers. Children who had all four factors were much more likely to have a recurrent febrile seizure than were those with none. Complex features were not associated with a higher recurrence risk. Overall, 30% had at least one recurrence, 17% had two recurrences, 9% had three recurrences, and 6% had more than three recurrences. Other factors identified in other studies included; abnormal developmental history, history of epilepsy in first-degree relatives, and attendance of day care. Most recurrences occurred within one year of the initial seizure. Among children who had one recurrence, younger age at the time of the first recurrence was the most important predictor of subsequent recurrences.

HOSPITAL ADMISSION & EVALUATION

It is generally accepted that hospital admission should be reserved for those with recurrent or prolonged complex seizures, with an underlying serious infection, or where parental anxiety and other social circumstances indicate. A brief period of observation may be indicated in a young febrile child with no clear focus of infection. However, routine hospital admission increases the tendency to perform unnecessary investigations and therefore should be discouraged. In the following section, we will discuss the indications, yield, and current recommendations regarding obtaining various investigations including blood studies, lumbar puncture, EEG, and neuroimaging in children with febrile seizures. The latest American Academy of Pediatrics (AAP) practice recommendations, which were based on reviewing 203 articles addressing the diagnostic evaluation of children with simple febrile seizures, will be highlighted. Overall, pediatricians are becoming more selective in admitting and investigating children with febrile seizures. The yield of investigations remains low and does not justify extensive work-up or prolonged hospitalization.

Laboratory Studies

It is not uncommon for children with simple febrile seizures to be subjected to various laboratory tests such as a complete blood count (CBC), serum electrolytes, calcium, phosphorous, magnesium, glucose, and urine or blood cultures. An underlying metabolic disorder presenting as a seizure in a febrile child is extremely uncommon as compared to those with afebrile seizures. The history and physical examination can direct the physician towards the underlying etiology. Infants with a history of vomiting, diarrhea, and altered fluid intake should have serum electrolyte profiles to exclude hypernatremia or hyponatremia, both of which may lead to seizures. Clinical evidence of dehydration and prolonged drowsiness or postictal obtundation are indications for measurement of serum electrolytes, blood sugar, calcium, and urea nitrogen. The yield of these tests, if done routinely, is very low. Despite these recommendations, a wide variation in physician evaluation and management persists. Sweeney et al, found marked variation in the number of investigations performed in each hospital of a regional population. Blood cultures and CBC were performed on 6-56% and 8-70% of children respectively and 23-78% were prescribed antibiotics. In another study, the risk of occult bacteremia was 2.1%, which is similar to those with fever alone. Other investigators who performed routine blood and urine cultures on all admitted children with febrile seizures found positive results in only 4.3% and 2.6% of the children respectively. Overall, the rates of bacteremia or serious bacterial illness were low and consistent with those published for febrile children without seizures.

LUMBAR PUNCTURE

Meningitis and meningo-encephalitis are the main concerns in a child presenting with fever and seizures. Seizures can be the presenting, but not the only feature, of up to 15% of children with meningitis. Although most infants (<18 months) who have seizures as an initial manifestation of meningitis do not have meningeal signs, they have other symptoms and findings that strongly suggest the correct diagnosis (*e.g.* altered state of consciousness, persistent vomiting, bulging fontanel, abnormal neurological signs). A thorough evaluation by an experienced clinician almost always will detect the child with meningitis. It is exceedingly rare for bacterial meningitis to be unsuspected clinically, only to be detected on the basis of routine evaluation of the CSF after a febrile seizure. The AAP recommends that LP be strongly considered in infants less than 12 months, considered in infants 12-18 months, and if clinically indicated in those greater than 18 months of age. It should also be strongly considered if the child had received prior oral antibiotics that may mask the clinical manifestations or results in transient improvement. Routine LP in all children with febrile convulsions is clearly not warranted. Others also concluded that excluding meningitis and encephalitis through careful history, examination, observation, and occasionally lumbar puncture in children less than 2 years of age, is all that is needed.

Electroencephalography (EEG)

The yield of routine EEG is low in neurologically normal children with febrile seizures even if the seizure is complex. We recently reported our prospective experience in 438 consecutive pediatric EEGs over a 1-year period. Overall, 6.5% had febrile seizures (including complex) and none had epileptiform discharges. Abnormal posterior slowing may occur shortly after the seizure and may be detected for as long as 10 days afterwards. This finding can serve to confirm the clinical impression that a seizure has occurred. However, EEG abnormalities are not predictive of recurrence or development of future epilepsy. This led to the conclusion that the routine practice of obtaining EEG in neurologically normal children with febrile seizures is not justified.

Neuroimaging (CT, MRI)

Neuroimaging with computed tomography (CT) or magnetic resonance imaging (MRI) should not be performed routinely. They should be considered in children with abnormal developmental history, abnormal head size, or focal neurological abnormalities. However, clinically important intracranial structural lesions are extremely uncommon in children with febrile seizures. Skull X-rays are not useful in investigating these children.

THERAPEUTIC INTERVENTIONS

Febrile seizures longer than 5-10 minutes should be treated actively. Airway, respiratory status, and circulatory status must be assessed. Blood should be obtained for electrolytes and glucose determination, if indicated. Antiepileptic drugs should be administered rectally or intravenously starting with lorazepam (0.1 mg/kg) or diazepam (0.3-0.5 mg/kg). If the seizure persists, an additional dose may be given. The child's respiratory status needs to be monitored carefully and intubation undertaken if the ventilatory status becomes compromised. Persistence of the seizure is rare. Rectal diazepam can also be used at home to treat febrile seizure recurrences of longer than 5 minutes. It is particularly useful in children at high risk for recurrent febrile status epilepticus or frequent repetitive febrile seizures. Parents can be taught to give the medication safely after providing an initial test dose under supervision. Antipyretics, such as acetaminophen and sponging with tepid water can help in reducing the body temperature. The role of prophylactic antipyretic and antiepileptic drugs in the management can be controversial. In the following section, we will discuss the indications, effectiveness, and current recommendations regarding various treatment modalities. The latest AAP practice recommendations, which were based on reviewing 300 articles addressing various therapeutic interventions of children with simple febrile seizures, will be highlighted.

Intermittent antipyretics

Treatment with antipyretics at the time of a febrile illness is helpful in providing comfort. The use of prophylactic antipyretics during a febrile illness is not effective in preventing recurrence of febrile seizures. Camfield et al in a randomized controlled trial compared recurrences in children who were given either phenobarbitone and antipyretics or antipyretics and placebo. The febrile seizure recurrence rate was 5% for the first group and 25% for the second group. In another study, neither moderate (10 mg/kg) nor did high (20 mg/kg) doses of acetaminophen alone reduce the incidence of recurrent febrile seizures.

Intermittent Diazepam

Intermittent rectal or oral diazepam given 3 times per day during a febrile illness has been proven effective in preventing febrile seizure recurrence. In a randomized controlled trial, oral diazepam (0.33 mg/kg Q8hr for 2-3 days of a febrile illness) was as effective as continuous phenobarbitone in preventing recurrent febrile seizures with a 44% risk reduction per patient per year. This practice has not been widely used by pediatricians and neurologists for several of reasons. First, the seizures may occur before the fever is noticed. Adverse effects such as lethargy, drowsiness, and ataxia are troublesome. Finally diazepam may mask evolving clinical signs of meningitis. The AAP advised that this treatment is not generally recommended.

Continuous Antiepileptic Drugs

Carbamazepine and phenytoin have not been shown to be effective in preventing febrile seizure recurrences. In randomized controlled trials, both phenobarbitone and valproic acid were found effective in preventing febrile seizure recurrences. Daily phenobarbitone reduced the rate of subsequent febrile seizures from 25% to 8% per year. Only 4% of children on valproic acid as compared to 35% of controls had recurrent febrile seizures. However, the risks and potential side effects of phenobarbitone (sleepiness, hyperactivity, cognitive effects) and valproic acid (hepatotoxicity, pancreatitis, thrombocytopenia) outweigh their benefits. As well, there is no available data suggesting that the prevention of recurrent febrile seizures reduces the risk of developing epilepsy.

RELATIONSHIP TO EPILEPSY SYNDROMES

Febrile seizures are classified as a special (situation related) epilepsy syndrome, according to the International League Against Epilepsy (ILAE) classification system. Rarely, febrile seizures can evolve to, or become associated with, other epilepsy syndromes including; 1) generalized epilepsy with febrile seizures plus syndrome, 2) temporal lobe epilepsy (TLE) due to mesial temporal sclerosis (MTS), 3) hemiconvulsion hemiplegia syndrome, 4) hemiconvulsion hemiplegia epilepsy syndrome, or 5) severe myoclonic epilepsy of infancy. The recently described syndrome of generalized epilepsy with febrile seizures plus has been previously discussed in the genetics section. The development of TLE secondary to MTS will be discussed in detail in the next section. We will discuss the other 3 syndromes briefly. Prolonged status epilepticus with a marked unilateral predominance can be followed by a long lasting hemiplegia characterizing the hemiconvulsion hemiplegia syndrome (HH syndrome) described by Gastaut *et al.* After several years, partial epilepsy originating from the affected hemisphere gives rise to the hemiconvulsion hemiplegia epilepsy syndrome (HHE syndrome). Brain MRI is characteristic, with initial edematous swelling of one hemisphere followed by global atrophy, independent of any vascular territory. Affected children frequently have cognitive impairments and intractable epilepsy. With the development of effective medications and aggressive management of status epielpticus, these two syndromes are becoming very uncommon. Finally, febrile seizures can be the initial manifestation of severe myoclonic epilepsy of infancy (SMEI). Recurrent mixed seizures occur in the first year of life with developmental and cognitive deterioration. The EEG shows fast spike wave and multifocal epileptiform discharges. The seizures are intractable, although myoclonic seizures tend to disappear. The syndrome is rare with recent evidence suggesting a genetic etiology. *De novo* mutations of the neuronal sodium channel alpha-subunit gene (SCN1A) were described recently in seven isolated SMEI patients. This is similar to the mutations described in patients with generalized epilepsy with febrile seizures plus syndrome, suggesting a link between the two syndromes.

FUTURE EPILEPSY & MESIAL TEMPORAL SCLEROSIS

Epilepsy occurs more frequently in children with a history of febrile seizures than in the general population. In a normal child with a simple febrile seizure, the risk is 1-2.5%, which is slightly higher than the 0.5% risk in the general population. Factors that increase this risk include abnormal neurological development, complex febrile seizures (particularly focal), and family history of epilepsy. Neurological abnormalities and complex seizures were associated with 9.2% incidence of afebrile seizures by seven years of age. In another population based study in which children with febrile seizures were observed into adulthood, three risk factors for developing epilepsy were identified including; focal seizures, prolonged seizures, and repeated episodes within 24 hours during the same illness. The risk of developing recurrent partial epilepsy was 6-8%, 17-22%, and 49% in children with one, two, or three of these risk factors, respectively. One of the most controversial issues in epilepsy of temporal lobe origin is whether prolonged febrile seizures cause MTS and therefore predisposing to TLE. Retrospective studies from tertiary epilepsy centers report that patients with refractory TLE considered for surgery often have a history of prolonged febrile seizures. However, population based studies have failed to confirm this association, as have prospective studies of febrile seizures. Studies assessing hippocampal volume have found an association between a smaller hippocampus and a history of febrile seizures. Data are conflicting as to whether a correlation exists between the duration of epilepsy and the reduction in hippocampal volume. The possibility of hippocampal injury was assessed using MRI in infants with complex febrile seizures. Abnormalities were found in the children with prolonged focal seizures but not in those with generalized seizures. Several infants developed hippocampal atrophy on follow-up imaging. Although these observations suggest seizure related hippocampal injury, the possibility of preexisting lesions leading to susceptibility to injury could not be excluded. Patients presenting to an epilepsy clinic were prospectively questioned about febrile seizures. Febrile seizures were reported by 13% of the patients. TLE (25%) was more likely to be preceded by febrile seizures than by extra-temporal epilepsy (6%) or generalized epilepsy (11%). Long duration was the most common feature associated with TLE. In another study, 524 children with epilepsy starting after the first year of life were evaluated. Febrile seizures were present in 14% and complex features were associated with a younger age at onset. No evidence that focal or prolonged febrile seizures were associated with TLE was found. Three children had hippocampal atrophy on their initial MRI, but none had a history of febrile seizures. The authors concluded that febrile seizures do not appear to cause TLE and the association may represent an inherent susceptibility in some children who are predisposed to prolonged febrile seizures and epilepsy simultaneously. Another study linking febrile seizures and TLE described two families with familial febrile seizures. MRI was performed on family members free of seizures, with febrile seizures only, and febrile seizures with subsequent TLE. All subjects with febrile seizures only and six normal relatives showed asymmetry in hippocampal size with changes in the internal architecture of the hippocampal bodies suggesting that the subtle preexisting hippocampal abnormalities facilitated the febrile seizures and contributed to the development of subsequent hippocampal sclerosis. The hippocampal abnormalities did not appear to be a consequence of the febrile seizures. Finally, a controlled animal study examined the effects of prolonged febrile seizures on immature rats. Prolonged hyperthermia-induced seizures did not result in subsequent spontaneous seizures in adult rats. However, the experimental animals developed hippocampal seizures after administering systemic kainate indicating a lowered seizure threshold. An analogous situation may exist in humans. Individuals predisposed to developing epilepsy, by a variety of factors, may become symptomatic in later years after having their thresholds modified by febrile seizures in infancy. To conclude, researchers still need to address the longstanding controversy regarding the relationship between prolonged febrile seizures and MTS. Large, longitudinal, prospective, multicentered trials of children with prolonged febrile seizures may provide answers to this key clinical question.

COGNITIVE & BEHAVIORAL EFFECTS

Long-term neurological sequelae including cognitive and behavioral disorders are extremely uncommon following febrile seizures. Reports of such associations have been anecdotal and derived from biased populations consisting of children assessed in tertiary care settings. This may reflect preexisting abnormalities. Most reports of new deficits have occurred after complex or prolonged febrile seizures. However, population based studies do not corroborate these reports. In the National Collaborative Perinatal Project, approximately 5% of children had febrile seizures lasting >30 minutes. None of these children sustained permanent motor deficits or impaired mental development unless they developed epilepsy. Similar findings were noted in a long-term, controlled, population-based study from the United Kingdom. Children with preexisting neurological or developmental abnormalities were excluded. At 10 years of age, no differences were noted in measurements of academic and behavioral functions in children with simple, complex, or recurrent febrile seizures compared to controls.

SUMMARY

Febrile seizures are common events, affecting up to 5% of children between the ages of 6 months and 5 years. Most febrile seizures are brief, do not require any specific treatment or workup, and have benign prognoses. Excluding meningitis and encephalitis, through careful history, examination, observation, and occasionally lumbar puncture, is the most important task of management. Routine hospital admission increases the tendency to perform unnecessary investigations and should be discouraged. Admission should be reserved for recurrent or long complex seizures, underlying serious infection, or where parental anxiety and other social circumstances necessitate such admission. LP should be strongly considered in infants <12 months of age, considered at 12-18 months, and if clinically indicated in infants >18 months. EEG, blood studies, and neuroimaging should not be performed routinely. Neither intermittent nor continuous antiepileptic drug treatments are recommended. However, parental education and emotional support are of paramount importance in all cases to alleviate associated anxieties.

BIBLIOGRAPHY

Al-Khathlan NA, Jan MMS: Clinical Profile of Admitted Children with Febrile Seizures. Neurosciences 2005;10(1):30-33.
Jan MMS, Girvin JP: Febrile Seizures: Update and Controversies. Neurosciences 2004;9(4):235-242.
Jan MM, Bamaga AK. MCQs: Febrile Seizures. Neurosciences 2009;14:394-5.
Jan MM: Assessment of the Utility of Pediatric Electroencephalography. Seizure 2002;11(2):99-103.

CHAPTER 12

Meningitis & Encephalitis

Abstract: Infections of the meninges (meningitis) and the brain (encephalitis) needs to be identified and managed promptly in order to prevent associated morbidity and mortality. Symptoms and signs of raised intracranial pressure are frequently the initial features of meningitis caused by bacterial or viral infections. Encephalitis is more frequently caused by viral infections with features that include seizures, personality change, decreased consciousness, and focal neurological manifestations. As the infection progress, mixed features are frequently encountered (meningoencephalitis). In this chapter, an updated overview of meningitis and encephalitis in infants and children is presented.

Keywords: Meningitis, Encephalitis, Viral, Bacterial, Tuberculosis, Fungal, Seizures, Encephalopathy, Lumber puncture, Antibiotics.

ETIOLOGY

Although routine childhood immunization has significantly decreased the number of serious viral infections, they remain more common than bacterial infections. The most common viruses that cause meningitis and encephalitis are listed in Table **1** and include enteroviruses, herpes simplex virus, and arboviruses. In clinical practice, the causative virus cannot be identified in up to 70% of cases. This is not the case for bacterial infections unless the patient received prior oral antibiotic therapy. The causative bacterial organisms vary with age as shown in Table **1**. Other infections causing meningoencephalitis in children, including fungal, are less common in immune competent patients.

Table 1: Common causes of meningitis and encephalitis in children.

Infection	Organisms
Viral	Enteroviruses
	Herpes simplex virus
	Myxoviruses (influenza, measles)
	Arboviruses
	Retroviruses (HIV)
	Rhabdoviruses (rabies)
Bacterial	
Newborn (early onset)	Escherichia coli
Newborn (late onset)	Group B streptococcus
Infants	Escherichia coli
School age	Group B streptococcus
	Enterococci
	Gram negative enteric bacilli (Pseudomonas and Klebsiella)
	Listeria monocytogenes
	Streptococcus pneumonia
	Neisseria meningitides
	Haemophilus influenza
	Streptococcus pneumonia
	Neisseria meningitides
	Mycobacterium tuberculosis
Fungal	Candida
	Cryptococcus neoformans
	Dimorphic Forms
	Blastomyces dermatitidis
	Coccidioides immitis
	Histoplasma capsulatum
	Aspergillus

VIRAL INFECTIONS

Aseptic Meningitis

Viral meningitis is a benign, self-limited disease from which most children recover completely. The term "aseptic" implies the presence of meningismus and cerebrospinal fluid (CSF) leukocytosis without bacterial or fungal infection. Enteroviruses are responsible for most cases, however, nonviral causes could be considered including Lyme disease, Kawasaki disease, leukemia, systemic lupus erythematosus, migraine, and drugs. In viral infections, the onset of symptoms is abrupt and characterized by fever, headache, and stiff neck, except in infants who do not have meningismus because of their open fontanels and sutures. Irritability, lethargy, and vomiting are common. The CSF contains 10-200 leukocytes/mm3, which are primarily lymphocytic. The protein concentration ranges between 50-100 mg/dL with normal glucose. Bacterial meningitis cannot be ruled out at the onset; therefore antibiotic therapy is indicated routinely until the CSF culture is negative. This is especially true for children who received prior oral antibiotic therapy. Treatment of herpes encephalitis with acyclovir is also indicated at the onset until the diagnosis is excluded (see next section). Otherwise, treatment of viral aseptic meningitis is symptomatic. Bed rest, quiet environment, and mild analgesics provide symptomatic relief. The acute illness usually lasts less than 1 week, but malaise and headache may continue for several weeks.

ENCEPHALITIS

Herpes Simplex virus (HSV) is the most serious treatable etiology of encephalitis. Other causative viruses are listed in Table **1** and are less common. HSV encephalitis accounts for 10-20% of cases with an estimated annual incidence of 2.3 cases per million population. HSV-1 (orofacial) is the causative agent of acute encephalitis (usually focal) after the neonatal period and HSV-2 (genital) is the causative agent of encephalitis (usually diffuse) in the newborn. In HSV-1, the initial orofacial infection may be asymptomatic. The virus replicates in the skin, infecting nerve fiber endings with retrograde neuronal infection reaching the olfactory or trigeminal ganglia. Further replication occurs within the ganglia before the virus enters a latent stage. Reactivation occurs during times of stress or acute illness. The reactivated virus ordinarily retraces its neural migration to the facial skin but occasionally spreads proximally to the brain, causing focal encephalitis predominantly affecting the temporal lobe (coming from the trigeminal ganglia) or inferior frontal lobe (coming from the olfactory ganglia). An immunocompromised state results in frequent reactivation and a more severe widespread infection. Clinically, the patient develops acute symptoms including fever, headache, lethargy, behavioral changes, nausea, and vomiting. Most children (80%) develop focal neurological signs including, hemiparesis, cranial nerve deficits, visual field loss, aphasia, and seizures. In HSV-2 infection the picture is more of a diffuse meningoencephalitis. The neonate acquires such a primary infection from the mother's genital tract. The initial clinical features are similar to those of aseptic meningitis caused by other viruses. CSF examination reveals pleocytosis with cell count within the 100s (up to 1000/mm3). Up to 500 red blood cells/mm3 may be present. The CSF protein concentration is usually high (80-100 mg/dL) with normal glucose. The identification of the organism in the CSF by polymerase chain reaction (PCR) has eliminated the need for brain biopsy to establish the diagnosis. Electroencephalography (EEG) demonstrates characteristic periodic lateralizing epileptiform discharges as the infection progress. However, MRI is a more sensitive early indicator of herpes encephalitis showing increased signal intensity involving the cortex and white matter in the temporal or inferior frontal lobes. Intravenous acyclovir treatment for both HSV-1 and HSV-2 infections is indicated for 2-3 weeks. Early treatment decreases the mortality rate from 70% in untreated patients to 30%. The highest mortality rate is in patients already in coma at treatment onset. Long term neurological complications are common and function returns to normal in only 40% of patients.

BACTERIAL INFECTIONS

Neonatal Meningitis

Meningitis occurs in approximately 1:2000 term newborns and accounts for 4% of all neonatal deaths. It is a consequence of septicemia and maternal infection is the main risk factor. Early-onset (first 5 days) and late-onset (after 5 days) patterns of meningitis have been identified. In early-onset neonatal meningitis, acquisition of infection occurs at the time of delivery, and the responsible organisms are usually Escherichia coli or group B streptococcus (Table 1). The newborn becomes symptomatic during the first week, and the mortality rate is 20-50%. In late-onset meningitis, acquisition of infection is postnatal, and the symptoms usually begin after the first week of life. Newborns requiring intensive care are specifically at risk of late-onset meningitis because of multiple instrumentations. Other organisms may be responsible including enterococci, gram negative enteric bacilli, and Listeria monocytogenes (Table 1). The mortality rate is 10-20%. Clinical features of both infection patterns include fever, hypothermia, jaundice, hepatomegaly, lethargy, irritability, feeding difficulties, seizures, respiratory distress, and subsequent apnea and shock. Bulging fontanels occurs in only 25% of neonates. The diagnosis should be confirmed by examination of the CSF. However, even in the absence of infection, the CSF of febrile newborns averages 11 leukocytes/mm3 (range 0–20), of which less than 6% are polymorphonuclear leukocytes. The protein concentration range is 40-130 mg/dL, and the glucose concentration range is 36-56 mg/dL. In newborns with meningitis, the leukocyte count is usually in the thousands, and the protein concentration is high. A Gram-stained smear of the CSF permits identification of an organism in up to 50% of cases. Rapid detection of bacterial antigens by immunoelectrophoresis, latex agglutination, and radioimmunoassays is helpful in the diagnosis of several bacteria. The choice of initial antibiotic therapy includes ampicillin and an aminoglycoside. An alternative regimen is ampicillin and cefotaxime. Identification of a specific organism leads to a more specific therapy. The duration of treatment for neonatal meningitis is at least 2 weeks beyond the time the CSF becomes sterile. CSF culture should be repeated after discontinuing antibiotic therapy. A positive culture indicates the need for a second course of therapy. Permanent neurological complications occur in 30-50% of survivors and include hydrocephalus, cerebral palsy, epilepsy, mental retardation, and deafness. The type of infecting organism and the gestational age are the main variables that determine mortality. Mortality rates are 20-30% and are highest for gram-negative infections.

Meningitis in Infants and Young Children

For children 6 weeks to 3 months old, group B streptococcus remains a leading cause of meningitis, and E coli is less common. Important organisms after 3 months of age include Streptococcus pneumonia, Neisseria meningitides and Haemophilus influenza (Table 1). However, Haemophilus influenza is becoming less common in many countries because of routine immunization. The onset of meningitis may be insidious or fulminating. Typical clinical features include fever, irritability, headache, vomiting, and lethargy. Seizures occur in around 30% of children. Examination reveals a sick and irritable child who resists being touched or moved. A bulging fontanel is a feature in young infants; however, papilledema is rarely seen. Petechial or hemorrhagic rash is seen in most children with meningococcemia. Meningeal irritation causes neck stiffness, characterized by limited mobility and pain on attempted flexion of the head. Focal neurological signs are unusual except in tuberculous meningitis or in complicated cases (*e.g.* abscess). Initial investigations include complete blood count showing leukocytosis with increased immature granulocytes. CSF examination is essential for the diagnosis and should be performed as quickly as possible when meningitis is suspected. Routine neuroimaging before lumbar puncture can result in significant diagnostic delays and therefore should be discouraged. Generalized increased intracranial pressure is always part of acute bacterial meningitis and is not a contraindication to lumbar puncture. The characteristic CSF findings include an increased pressure, cloudy appearance, polymorphonuclear leukocytosis (thousands), decreased glucose (<50% of plasma), increased protein, positive gram stain and culture. The CSF abnormalities may vary according to the type of organism, the timing of the lumbar puncture, the previous use of antibiotics, and the immunocompetence of the host. Cultures of the blood, urine, and nasopharynx are also indicated. The diagnosis of the syndrome of inappropriate antidiuretic hormone secretion requires measurement of serum electrolytes and requires careful fluid management. Every child at risk of tuberculous meningitis requires a tuberculin skin test. Antibiotic therapy should be given immediately and should not be delayed until the CSF results are obtained. Vancomycin and a third-generation cephalosporin are recommended initially. The final choice awaits the results of culture and antibiotic sensitivity. The response to treatment and outcome depends on the infecting organism and the speed of initiating therapy. Rapid decline of neurological function is indicative of the severity of cerebral edema and cerebral vasculitis. Peripheral vascular collapse can result from brainstem herniation, endotoxic shock, or adrenal failure. Up to 10% of the survivors develop sensory neural hearing loss. The incidence of hearing loss is highest with S pneumoniae infection (30%). Identification of hearing loss and early rehabilitation will lessen the long-term educational and social difficulties these children may experience. Some children (4%) have other long term neurological deficits.

Meningitis in School-Age Children

S pneumoniae and N meningitidis account for most cases of bacterial meningitis in previously healthy school-age children, whereas Mycobacterium tuberculosis is a leading cause of meningitis in economically deprived populations (Table **1**). The symptoms do not differ substantially from those encountered in preschool children. Predisposing conditions include otitis media, complement deficiency, sickle cell disease, asplenia, and chronic illnesses. Patients at high risk require immunization with pneumococcal and meningococcal vaccines. Vancomycin and a third-generation cephalosporin are usually recommended for treatment. Penicillin G and ampicillin are equally effective in treating penicillin-sensitive strains of S pneumoniae. A 2-day course of oral rifampin is prescribed for all household contacts. Up to 8% of children treated for bacterial meningitis develop major neurological deficits (*e.g.* mental retardation, seizures, hydrocephalus, cerebral palsy, blindness, hearing loss). Learning difficulties are more commonly encountered in these patients (up to 18%) as they grow older.

Recurrent Bacterial Meningitis

Recurrence usually is caused by a different bacterial pathogen; however infection by the same organism is considered a recurrence if it occurs more than three weeks after the completion of initial therapy. Patients at risk of recurrence include those with a history of skull base injury or CSF leak. Other causes include congenital tracts and immunodeficiency. Bacteria can migrate into the subarachnoid space along congenital or acquired pathways from the skull or spinal dural defects. Meningitis can be the sole symptom and is caused by bacteria normally present in the paranasal sinuses, gut, or skin surface. Streptococcus pneumoniae is common with cranial dural lesions while staphylococci are found in cases with cutaneous association and gram negative rods are found in cases with enteric association. Examples of congenital anatomical defects include encephaloceles, skull fractures, neurenteric cyst, fibrous dysplasia, persistent craniopharyngeal duct, and lumbosacral defects. Dural lesions can also be acquired following trauma, surgery, inflammation (osteomyelitis), tumors, or increased CSF pressure. High-resolution computed tomography, fluorescein endoscopy, cisternography, and magnetic resonance imaging can be all used to diagnose these rare causes of recurrent meningitis and guide the provision of the necessary surgical repair. If all the imaging studies are negative, immunological studies should be performed to exclude an underlying immune deficiency syndrome.

Tuberculous Meningitis

Worldwide, tuberculosis (TB) remains a leading cause of morbidity and death in children. It occurs with a higher frequency in developing countries and where sanitation is poor or with overcrowding. However, tuberculosis accounts for only 5% of bacterial meningitis in developed countries. The peak incidence of tuberculous meningitis is between 6 months and 2 years of age. Infection follows inhalation of the organism from infected contacts. Within 6 months, pulmonary tuberculosis disseminates to other organs, including the brain. The first symptoms tend to be more insidious than with other bacterial meningitides, however, a fulminant course is occasionally seen. TB meningitis, in contrast to fungal meningitis, is not a cause of chronic meningitis. If not treated, a child with TB meningitis dies within few weeks. Most often, fever develops first, and the child becomes listless, irritable with vomiting and abdominal pain. Headache and vomiting become increasingly frequent and severe. Signs of meningismus develop during the second week after onset of fever. Cerebral infarction occurs in one third of affected children. Seizures are common and the consciousness level declines progressively with focal neurological deficits including, cranial neuropathies and hemiparesis. The diagnosis should be considered in any child with a household contact. General use of tuberculin skin testing in children at risk is crucial to early detection. The peripheral white blood cell count generally is elevated with associated hyponatremia and hypochloremia as a result of inappropriate antidiuretic hormone secretion. The CSF is usually cloudy with high leukocyte count, predominantly lymphocytic. CSF glucose declines and the protein increases steadily throughout the illness. Smears of CSF stained by the acid-fast technique generally show the bacillus. Recovery of the organism from the CSF is not always successful, even when guinea pig inoculation is used. Newer diagnostic tests include PCR, enzyme-linked immunosorbent assay, and radioimmunoassay tests for antimycobacterial antigens with reported sensitivities reaching 75%. Early treatment enhances the prognosis for survival and neurological recovery. Isoniazid, streptomycin, rifampin, and pyrazinamide are recommended for 2 months. Isoniazid and rifampin should be continued for an additional 10 months. Corticosteroids can be used initially to reduce inflammation and cerebral edema. Communicating hydrocephalus is a common complication of because of impaired CSF absorption. Complete neurological recovery is unlikely when the child becomes comatose with mortality rates reaching 20%, even with early treatment.

FUNGAL INFECTIONS

Fungal infections of the central nervous system may cause acute, subacute, or chronic meningitis, in addition to abscesses and granulomas. Candida and Cryptococcus infections are the most common, followed by Coccidioides, Aspergillus, and Zygomycetes (Table 1). Candida is a common inhabitant of the mouth and intestinal tract. Ordinarily it causes no symptoms; however, Candida can multiply and become an important pathogen in children with immunosuppression, prolonged antibiotic use, debilitating diseases, transplant recipients, and critically ill children undergoing treatment with long-term vascular catheters. Candidal meningitis is extremely uncommon in healthy non-hospitalized children. Candida reaches the brain by vascular dissemination and the brain is involved less often than other organs. Fever, lethargy, and vomiting are the prominent features. Hepatosplenomegaly and arthritis may be present. As the infection progress, meningismus, papilledema, and seizures occurs leading to decreased level of consciousness. The organism can be isolated from the CSF or blood. The CSF shows a predominantly neutrophilic response with increased protein and mild decrease of the glucose concentration. Children with a candidal abscess rather than meningitis may have near-normal CSF results. CT reveals a mass lesion resembling a pyogenic abscess or tumor. Indwelling vascular catheters should be removed and the patient treated with amphotericin B and flucytosine for 6-12 weeks.

CONCLUSIONS

Despite the availability of modern therapies, meningitis and encephalitis remain potentially life threatening infections with significant morbidity. Routine childhood immunization has significantly decreased the number of serious infections. However, this remains problematic in developing countries where immunization rates are suboptimal. The most common viruses include enteroviruses, herpes simplex virus, and arboviruses. The causative bacterial organisms vary with age and fungal infections are less common in immune competent patients. CSF examination is essential for the diagnosis and should be performed as quickly as possible. Routine neuroimaging before lumbar puncture can result in significant diagnostic delays and therefore should be discouraged. The CSF abnormalities may vary according to the type of organism, the timing of the lumbar puncture, the previous use of antibiotics, and the immunocompetence of the host. Every child at risk of tuberculous meningitis requires a tuberculin skin test. Antibiotic therapy should be given immediately and should not be delayed until the CSF results are obtained. The final choice awaits the results of culture and antibiotic sensitivity. The response to treatment and outcome depends on the infecting organism and the speed of initiating therapy. Major neurological deficits develop in 8% of children and up to 18% may have future learning difficulties.

BIBLIOGRAPHY

Al-Khathlan NA, Jan MMS: Clinical Profile of Admitted Children with Febrile Seizures. Neurosciences 2005;10(1):30-33.
Jan MMS, Girvin JP: Febrile Seizures: Update and Controversies. Neurosciences 2004;9(4):235-242.
Jan MMS, Al-Buhairi AR, Baeesa SS: Concise Outline of the Nervous System Examination for the Generalist. Neurosciences 2001;6(1):16-22.
Jan MM. Meningitis and encephalitis in infants and children. Saudi Med J 2012;33(1):11-16.

CHAPTER 13

Infant Hypotonia

Abstract: Hypotonia in infants and children can be a confusing clinical presentation, which often leads to unnecessary investigations. Stepwise and accurate assessment is very important to reach the correct diagnosis. Although specific treatments are not always available, accurate diagnosis is critical to predict the clinical course, associated manifestations, complications, prognosis, and provide genetic counseling. In this chapter, I present a concise clinical approach for evaluating the hypotonic infant. Some practical tips and skills are discussed to improve the likelihood of obtaining accurate diagnosis.

Keywords: Infant, Hypotonia, Weakness, Myopathy, Dystrophy, Fasiculations, Areflexia, EMG, Muscle biopsy, Rehabilitation.

DEFINITION & CLASSIFICATION

Muscle tone is defined as resistance to passive movement. Muscle tone develops in an orderly sequence through gestation and continues to change after birth. Increased muscle extensibility and passivity characterize infantile hypotonia. Hypotonia can be global, truncal, or predominantly involving the limbs. Hypotonia can result from a variety of central or peripheral causes (Table **1**). Therefore, hypotonia is a phenotype of many clinical conditions with variable prognosis. Central hypotonia results from global brain dysfunction due to toxic, metabolic, or hypoxic insult. Certain drugs, such as barbiturates and benzodiazepines, can be implicated. As well, congenital or developmental brain abnormalities can cause central hypotonia. Down, Prader-Willi, and Smith-Lemli-Opitz syndromes are important examples. On the other hand, focal brain pathology usually results in hypertonia depending on the site and extent of the lesion (*e.g.* hemiplegia, diplegia, quadriplegia). It is important recognize that hypotonia is not equivalent to weakness. Infants with central causes, such as Down syndrome, may have severe hypotonia and normal muscle strength. Peripheral hypotonia is frequently associated with weakness and results from a lesion involving the peripheral nervous system (anterior horn cell, roots, nerves, neuromuscular junction, or muscles). Hypotonia with weakness due to a peripheral nervous system lesion can be predominantly distal (neuropathic) or proximal (myopathic). The distinction between central and peripheral hypotonia is critical for proper evaluation and management as shown in Table **1**. In general, central hypotonia is much more commonly encountered in general pediatric and neurology practices than peripheral hypotonia. Mixed hypotonia occurs when primarily central disorders present with both profound hypotonia and weakness, particularly in the neonatal period. They include Prader-Willi syndrome and acute conditions such as hemorrhage or infarction of the deep central gray matter of the brain or spinal cord. As well, combined central and peripheral abnormalities can present with hypotonia and weakness. Examples include congenital muscular dystrophy, congenital myotonic dystrophy, cervical spinal cord injury, acid maltase deficiency, and some mitochondrial and peroxisomal disorders. Note that conditions such as Ehlers-Danlos syndrome or osteogenesis imperfecta can also present with hypotonia. In these disorders, hypotonia results from ligamentous laxity, rather than a neurological abnormality.

HISTORY TAKING

Detailed history is critical in the evaluation of the hypotonic infant. The usual presenting complaint in these infants is motor delay rather than hypotonia *per se*. The distinction between a static (brain insults, congenital structural myopathies) or progressive (spinal muscular atrophy and dystrophies) course is critical. Static causes usually results in slow improvements and developmental gains, while progressive causes results in relentless deterioration. Perinatal history may provide information that supports the diagnosis. Infants with a peripheral neuromuscular disorder may have history of polyhydramnios (due to decreased fetal swallowing), decreased fetal movements, and malpresentation. History of birth trauma, asphyxia, or infection may predispose to central hypotonia. However, note that infants with congenital neuromuscular disorders may be less able to tolerate the stress associated with labor and delivery and thus, be more susceptible to birth depression. Seizures, cognitive dysfunction, vision or hearing impairment points towards a central etiology. A family history of neuromuscular abnormalities may be informative because many disorders are inherited. Examples of familial neuromuscular diseases include congenital myotonic dystrophy, spinal muscular atrophy, metabolic disorders (*e.g.* mitochondrial disease, acid maltase deficiency, defects of creatine synthesis).

Table 1: Summary of the types of hypotonia.

CENTRAL HYPOTONIA
Site of Lesion: Brain, brainstem, spinal cord (above the origin of the cranial nerve nuclei or anterior horn cells).
Causes: Brain malformations, chromosomal aberration: *e.g.* Down's syndrome, Prader-Willi syndrome, cerebellar hypoplasia.
Clues to Diagnosis: Histoy of brain insult, seizures, dysmorphic features, lack of interest to the surroundings, abnormal head size, normal spontaneous movements, normal or increased reflexes, persistence of primitive reflexes, organomegaly.

PERIPHERAL HYPOTONIA
Site of Lesion: Cranial nerve nuclei, anterior horn cell, nerve roots, peripheral nerves, neuromuscular junction or muscle.
Causes: Spinal cord injury, spinal muscular atrophy, poliomyelitis, peripheral neuropathy, Guillain-Barre syndrome, myasthenia gravis, infantile botulism, congenital or metabolic myopathy, muscular dystrophy.
Clues to Diagnosis: Decreased fetal movements, alertness and responsiveness, weakness with little spontaneous movements, absent or decreased reflexes, fasiculations, muscle atrophy, and sensory loss.

MIXED HYPOTONIA
Features of both central and peripheral hypotonia due to combined central and peripheral pathology (*e.g.* peroxisomal, lysosomal, and mitochondrial disorders, or any cause of peripheral hypotonia with an acquired brain insult)

ASSESSMENT OF MUSCLE TONE

Hypotonia can be identified readily by inspection. In the normal term infant, both the upper and lower limbs have predominantly flexor tone with active limb movements. Normal muscle tone is decreased in the premature compared to the term infant. Flexor tone in premature infants diminishes with decreasing gestational age. Limb tone is examined by assessing the passive mobility in at least three joints in each limb (*e.g.* shoulder, elbow, wrist). Each joint is moved in all ranges of motion in a rapid manner and compared to the other side. Hand shaking is a useful initial step in an older child. Another useful maneuver is gentle shaking of both hands and feet to assess symmetry of the muscle tone. In the lower limb, rolling the leg (internal and external rotation at the hip) while the child is lying supine in bed, is easy and useful to assess more proximal tone. Before concluding the findings, truncal tone should be assessed. Pulling the infant from supine to sitting position results in a slight head lag at term. No head lag should be seen normally by the age of 3 months. The hypotonic infant lies supine in a frog leg position with the hips flexed and abducted. Holding the infant in horizontal (ventral) suspension is accompanied by flexion of the limbs, straightening the back, and maintaining the head in the body plane for a few seconds. By age 3 months, the head can be raised above the body plane momentarily on ventral suspension. Holding the infant under the arms identifies truncal resistance that allows the infant to be easily supported without slipping through the examiner's hands. Finally, it is important to evaluate the mother's muscle strength and tone to exclude myotonia (delayed muscle relaxation). This is usually tested by asking the mother to close her eyes tightly or make a tight fist then quickly opening it. This can be an important clue to congenital myotonic dystrophy.

PHYSICAL EXAMINATION

Careful general examination is needed. Abnormalities of respiratory rate, pattern, or diaphragmatic movement can accompany congenital myopathies. Dysmorphic features and congenital defects points towards a central etiology. Weight, length, and head circumference should be measured and plotted on percentile charts. Abnormal head size (micro or macrocephaly) suggest a central cause (Table 1). Pallor and bruising could suggest an acute traumatic etiology. The skin should also be carefully examined to exclude neurocutaneous syndromes or dermatomyositis. Examination of the back is critical in children with paraplegia to exclude spina bifida. The most important step in initial neurological examination is to differentiate between an upper and lower motor neuron lesion. Abnormal eye fixation or follow suggests a lesion above the level of the brainstem. Facial diplegia occurs in some neuromuscular disorders (*e.g.* congenital myotonic dystrophy). It also can be associated with severe acute basal ganglia damage (*e.g.* mitochondrial disease, Leigh disease). The infant's ability to suck and swallow should be assessed. Difficulty with swallowing may lead to drooling. The character of the cry should be noted, and the tongue should be examined for fasciculations, which typically are associated with spinal muscular atrophy. However, they can be seen with hypoglossal motor nerve dysfunction accompanying glycogen storage diseases, hypoxic-ischemic encephalopathy, and infantile neuroaxonal degeneration. Motor examination identifies the extent and distribution of hypotonia (limb, truncal, or global). By inspection, good level of alertness and little spontaneous movements suggest peripheral hypotonia. Spontaneous fisting or an abnormal primitive reflex in response to handling suggests cerebral dysfunction. Peripheral hypotonia is associated with weakness with decreased spontaneous movements. Most neuropathies (except spinal muscular atrophy) results in distal weakness. On the other hand, most myopathies (except myotonic dystrophy) results in proximal weakness. Central hypotonia is usually associated with reasonable power. Hypotonia can be a non-localizing initial motor presentation of a brain insult that may later evolve to hemiplegia, quadriplegia, or diplegia. In these cases neonatal hypotonia is followed by motor delay and subsequent spasticity. Spasticity replaces neonatal hypotonia in children with cerebral palsy towards the end of the first year of life as myelination progress. Contractures are mainly found in infants with peripheral nerve or muscle involvement. Deep tendon reflexes may help distinguish between upper and lower motor neuron lesions. Abnormally brisk reflexes with clonus suggest central involvement, whereas absent reflexes are consistent with a neuropathic lesion or severe myopathy. Sensations should be tested as sensory loss suggests peripheral neuropathy. Other system examination may provide important clues to the diagnosis. Hepatomegaly and/or splenomegaly are evident in the neurovisceral sphingolipidosis, mucopolysaccharidosis, peroxisomal, and mitochondrial disorders. Cardiomyopathy may suggest muscular dystrophy, carnitine deficiency, or fatty acid oxidation disorders. Features of renal failure are evident in Lowe syndrome.

INVESTIGATIONS

The required investigations depend on the findings on history and physical examination. Many times, the etiology is apparent and no further tests are needed. Important blood tests include muscle enzymes and thyroid function tests. Serum creatine kinase level is normal in central and neuropathic causes. It is mildly elevated in myopathies (100s) and markedly elevated in muscular dystrophies (1000s), as will be discussed in the next chapter. Cardiac assessment including echocardiography is needed in muscular dystrophy to exclude cardiac involvement. Neuroimaging, particularly MRI, is needed in children with central hypotonia to exclude brain anomalies, degenerative disorders or acquired lesions. Electrodiagnostic studies include needle electromyography (EMG) and nerve conduction studies. This test is difficult to conduct reliably in young infants and uncooperative patients. As well, the results are not specific. It can show denervation changes in spinal muscular atrophy and peripheral neuropathy. Myopathic changes are expected in myopathies or dystrophies. Therefore, EMG is sensitive but not specific. Other authors also stressed the controversy over the usefulness of EMG in the assessment of the hypotonic infant even if neuromuscular disease is suspected. Accurate clinical evaluation can replace this test with emphasis on more specific tests, such as muscle biopsy in peripheral hypotonia and brain MRI in central hypotonia. If myasthenia gravis is suspected, tensilon test is recommended. In muscular disorders, it is important to differentiate between myopathies and dystrophies (next chapter). Muscle biopsy is the gold standard for diagnosing muscle diseases. Avoid taking the sample from a mildly involved muscle, because it may not reveal the pathology. As well, avoid severely involved muscles that may be fibrotic and not reveal the characteristic findings. Finally, avoid sampling a muscle that was recently needled for EMG because of post traumatic inflammatory changes that may confuse the picture. Muscle biopsy can also help in some neuropathies such as spinal muscular atrophy showing group atrophy. However, note that many causes of hypotonia are central in origin and therefore a muscle biopsy is not needed. Recently, DNA study for the specific genetic defect has replaced the need to do the invasive biopsy in some disorders, such as spinal muscular atrophy. Rapid molecular diagnosis is also now possible for congenital muscular dystrophies, several forms of congenital myopathies, and congenital myotonic dystrophy. Genetic tests are helpful when positive, however, muscle biopsy is indicated if the DNA testing is negative (false negative). Reaching a specific diagnosis is very important for providing appropriate therapy, prognosis, and genetic counseling. When possible, prenatal diagnosis can be offered in subsequent pregnancies.

MANAGEMENT

Hypotonia is an expression of many disorders involving the central and peripheral nervous system. Once the correct diagnosis is confirmed, specific treatments can be offered. The diagnosis of benign congenital hypotonia should be made only after excluding common etiologies. The disorder is rare with isolated hypotonia that recovers completely before 2 years of age. Some studies have shown that some of these children may have additional motor deficits on long term follow-up. Central hypotonia and hypotonia secondary to congenital myopathy usually improves with time. The prognosis is worst for hypotonia secondary to neuronal pathology or other progressive central disorders. Treatment is directed towards the underlying etiology, clinical manifestations, or complications of the disease. Some central causes are correctable neurosurgicaly such as hydrocephalus and posterior fossa arachnoid cyst. If the hypotonia is drug related, removing the drug is curative. However, frequently it is multifactorial. Some metabolic myopathies are correctable by specific treatments to counteract the offending metabolite, replace the dysfunctional enzyme, or vitamin therapy. Example is the use of dichloroacetate, L-carnitine, and Coenzyme Q10 in mitochondrial disorders, and the reduction of phytanic acid intake in refsum disease. Significant advances have also been made in regards to specific treatment of various metabolic encephalopathies resulting in central hypotonia. Pediatricians and neonatologists must be vigilant in early detection as early diagnosis and intervention is crucial to avoid CNS sequelae and death. Treatment is also directed towards treatable complications such as epilepsy, sleep disorder, behavioral symptoms, feeding difficulties, skeletal deformities, and recurrent chest infections. These children require a multidisciplinary team approach with the involvement of several specialties including pediatrics, neurology, genetics, orthopedics, physiotherapy, and occupational therapy. Physiotherapy is mainly preventative to avoid contractures and wasting, but will not increase muscle tone. Occupational therapy is more important in terms of seating and mobility. Counseling the families about potentially preventable disorders is very important in the management of these children. Consanguinity needs to be strongly discouraged in order to prevent inherited causes in our region.

BIBLIOGRAPHY

Jan MMS: The Hypotonic Infant: Clinical Approach. J Pediatr Neurol 2007;5(3):181-7.

CHAPTER 14

Muscle Weakness

Abstract: Weakness is a common presentation of a wide variety of central and peripheral nervous system disorders. Weakness can be due to an organic CNS lesion or due to pseudoparalysis secondary to pain. Weakness due to brain lesion usually takes the distribution according to the site and extent of the lesion (*e.g.* hemiplegia, diplegia, quadriplegia). Weakness due to peripheral nervous system lesion can be predominantly distal (neuropathic) or proximal (myopathic). The approach to a child presenting with acute or chronic weakness is presented in this chapter.

Keywords: Muscle, Weakness, Hypotonia, Paralysis, Myasthenia, EMG, Myopathy, Neuropathy, Dystrophy, Muscle biopsy, Physiotherapy.

HISTORY

A number of features and characteristics of the weakness can point towards the underlying diagnosis. Important features of the weakness include:

- Acute (Guillain-Barre syndrome) or chronic (myopathies)

- Progressive (dystrophies), static, or improving

- Distal (neuropathic) or Proximal (myopathic)

- Ascending (*e.g.* Guillain-Barre syndrome)

- Diurnal variation (myasthenia gravis)

- Bulbar symptoms (polio)

- Sensory symptoms (neuropathic)

Preceding upper respiratory tract infection, chicken pox, measles, and infectious mononucleosis could suggest a post-infectious GBS or ADEM. Back pain or muscle pain, which increases by cough, sneezing, or movement of the spine, could suggest a spinal inflammatory process. Exclude symptoms of urine or stool incontinence. Symptoms of increased intracranial pressure suggest a central cause. History of trauma, drug intake, or recent vaccination can give hints towards the underlying etiology.

EXAMINATION

In the general examination, look for associated skin rash that can be the result of dermatomyositis. Always examine the back in children with paraplegia to exclude spina bifida. The most important step in initial neurological examination is to differentiate between an upper and lower motor neuron lesion (Table **1**). Most neuropathies (except spinal muscular atrophy) results in distal weakness. On the other hand, most myopathies (except myotonic dystrophy) results in proximal weakness. Weakness due to brain insult can take the form of hemiplegia, monoplegia, quadriplegia, double hemiplegia, or triplegia. In hemiplegia, the arm is typically more affected than the leg. This is because of larger cortical representation (motor homonculus) of the hand and arm compared to a smaller leg area. Diplegia is present when the lower extremities are primarily affected with milder involvement of the upper extremities. Monoplegia refers to single limb involvement. This is usually the result of very mild hemiplegia with arm deficits only. When all four limbs are involved, quadriplegia is the appropriate descriptive term. Double hemiplegia refers to the child with quadriplegia involving the arms more than the legs with side asymmetry. Triplegia is rare and usually results from milder and very asymmetric double hemiplegia (sparing one leg) or asymmetric diplegia (sparing one arm). Quadriplegia can be also the result of spinal cord lesion (poliomyelitis), neuropathy (Guillain-Barre syndrome), neuromuscular junction disorders (botulism, myasthenia gravis), or muscle involvement (myopathy, dystrophy). Paraplegia can be central (para-sagittal meningioma, sagittal sinus thrombosis) due to involvement of the leg area, or spinal due to compressive lesion, trauma, transverse myelitis, or rarely, vascular insult.

Table 1: Differentiation of upper and lower motor neuron lesions.

Feature	UMNL	LMNL
Site of the lesion	Cerebrum hemispheres, cerebellum, brain stem, or spinal cord	Anterior horn cell, roots, nerves, neuromuscular junction, or muscles
Muscle weakness	Quadriplegia, hemiplegia, diplegia, triplegia	Proximal (myopathy) Distal (neuropathy)
Muscle tone	Spasticity/Rigidity	Hypotonia
Fasiculations	Absent	Present (tongue)
Tendon reflexes	Hyperreflexia	Hypo/areflexia
Abdominal reflexes	Absent (depending on the involved spinal level)	Present
Sensory loss	Cortical sensations	Peripheral sensations
Electromyography (EMG)	Normal nerve conduction Decreased interference pattern and firing rate	Slow nerve conduction Large motor units Fasciculations and fibrillations

INVESTIGATIONS

The required investigations depend on the findings on history and physical examination. Many times, the etiology is apparent and no further tests are needed. Important blood tests include muscle enzymes, thyroid function tests, echocardiography, EMG, and muscle biopsy. Table **1** shows the differentiating features of upper and lower motor neuron lesions. Table **2** shows important differentiating features of myopathies and dystrophies. If myasthenia gravis is suspected, tensilon test is recommended (Table **3**). Muscle biopsy is the gold standard for diagnosing muscle diseases. Avoid taking the sample from a mildly involved muscle, because it may not reveal the pathology. As well, avoid a severely involved muscle that may be fibrotic and not reveal the characteristic findings. Finally, avoid sampling a muscle that was recently needled for EMG because of post traumatic inflammatory changes that may confuse the picture. Muscle biopsy can also help in some neuropathies such as spinal muscular atrophy showing group atrophy. However, note that many causes of hypotonia are central in origin and therefore a muscle biopsy is not needed. Recently, DNA study for the specific genetic defect has replaced the need to do the invasive biopsy in some disorders, such as Duchenne muscular dystrophy. These tests are helpful when positive, however, muscle biopsy is indicated if the DNA testing is negative (false negative).

Table 2: Differentiating features of myopathies and dystrophies.

Feature	Myopathy	Dystrophy
Examples of disorders	Thyroid disease Centronuclear myopathy Central core disease	Duchenne Becker dystrophy Limb girdle
Etiology	Congenital Metabolic Endocrine	Genetic
Inheritance	Usually none Autosomal recessive	Always inherited
Progression	Static or improve with time or treatment	Always progressive
Muscle enzymes	Mildly increased (100s)	Markedly increased (1000s)
EMG	No fibrillations	Fibrillations because of active muscle necrosis

Table 3: Tensilon test for suspected Myasthenia Gravis.

Requirements:
1- Tensilon (Edrophonium hydrochloride), 10 mg/ml.
2- Resuscitation equipment.
3- 0.4 mg of injectable Atropine.
4- 10 ml syringe filled with normal saline.
5- Multiswitch stopcock (optional).
6- Videocamera (optional).
Dose:
0. 15 mg/kg (maximum 10 mg), action within 1 min and dissipate in 5-10 min.
Procedure (using a 10 mg dose):
1- Baseline assessment of weakness (+/- videorecording).
2- Inject 1 ml of normal saline and observe for 1 minute.
3- Inject 0.2 ml (2 mg) tensilon and flush tubing with 1ml saline (Test dose).
4- If no response, inject 0.8 ml (8 mg) and flush tubing with 1 ml saline.
Alternatives:
Intramuscular Neostigmine (Prostigmin), dose (mg) = <u>weight in kg</u> × 1.5   70   Pretreat with 0.4 mg I/M Atropine, 15 min before the test.   Effect in 30-45 minutes.

TREATMENT

Once the correct diagnosis is made, accurate treatment can be provided. IV immune globulins can be used acutely for a number of disorders, particularly Guillain-Barre syndrome (Table **4**). Treatment of the underlying etiology (tumor, infection) is needed. As well, treatment of associated manifestations and complications is required, such as cardiomyopathy, respiratory failure, and skeletal deformities. There is strong evidence that oral steroids (prednisolone) at 0.75 mg/kg/day given as a single morning dose can prolong ambulation and slow down the progression of Duchenne muscular dystrophy by at least 2 years. Once the child looses independent ambulation, the side effects of steroids outweigh their benefit. Newer steroids with fewer side effects are now available, such as deflazocort.

Table 4: Protocol for IV Immune Globulin (IVIG).

Initiation:
5% Gamma Globulin 2gm/kg (total dose), infusion rate at 0. 01-0. 02 ml/kg/min for 30 min then double the infusion rate every 30 min until a maximum rate of 0.06-0.08 ml/kg/min.
Monitoring:

Vital Signs (temperature, blood pressure, pulse, and respiration) at:
       - Baseline
       - Every 15 min for 1 hr
       - Every 30 min for 1 hr
       - Every 60 min for the remainder of infusion

Adverse Reactions:
Observe for the following adverse reactions, particularly during the first hour of infusion: Chills, fever, headache, vomiting, hypotension, malaise, chest tightness, disorientation, anxiety, wheezing, abdominal pain, myalgia, arthralgia, flushing, and skin rash.
Anaphylaxis:
For severe anaphylactic reaction, stop the infusion immediately. Have Epinephrine 1:1000 in the room. For mild reactions, reduce the infusion rate until symptoms subside.

BIBLIOGRAPHY

Jan MM. Cerebral palsy: comprehensive review and update. Ann Saudi Med 2006;26(2):123-132.

Al-Said YA, Al-Rached HS, Al-Qahtani HA, Jan MM: Severe Proximal Myopathy with Remarkable Recovery after Vitamin D Treatment. Can J Neurol Sci 2009;36(3):336-9.

Jan MM, Benstead TJ, Schwartz M: Electromyography Related Anxiety and Pain: A Prospective Study. Can J Neurol Sci 1999;26:294-297.

CHAPTER 15

Acute Hemiplegia

Abstract: Stroke is defined as a rapidly developing clinical signs of focal or global disturbance of cerebral functions with symptoms lasting 24 hr or longer or leading to death with no apparent cause other than of vascular origin. Childhood stroke is increasingly recognized with an incidence exceeding 3.3 in 100, 000 children per year, more than double the estimates from past decades. The risk factors for ischemic stroke in children are diverse and challenging. The most common cause of ischemic stroke in children is thrombotic vessel occlusion. Risk factors include prothrombin 20210G-A (PT20210) mutation, factor V Leiden 1691 G-A mutation, and hereditary deficiencies of protein S, protein C, and antithrombin III. Recently, another thrombophilic factor has been described, that is, an elevated level of factor VIII procoagulant activity. Cardio-embolic causes are amongst the most important to identify early in order to prevent recurrence. Spastic hemiplegia can also be an initial manifestation of a number of metabolic or degenerative disorders such as Metachromatic leukodystrophy, Adrenoleukodystrophy, Leigh disease, MELAS, Sneddon syndrome, Homocystinuria, Fabry disease, and Menkes disease. Finally, inherited dyslipidemic states can occur rarely in children resulting in atherosclerotic disease. Many of these disorders have a distinct inheritance patterns and specific defects. Establishing such specific diagnoses will be therefore extremely important for providing appropriate therapy, prognosis, and genetic counseling.

Keywords: Muscle, Weakness, Hypotonia, Paralysis, Hemiplegia, Stroke, Thrombosis, Embolism, MRA, Angiography, Physiotherapy.

EPIDEMIOLOGY

There are limited studies on pediatric stroke, and most of the available studies are retrospective. There is evidence that stroke incidence and prevalence are increasing. Based on population based studies, the rate increased from 2.5/100, 000 children/year in 1970 to 3.3/100, 000 children/year currently. The rate in Japan is 0.2, excluding moya moya disease. The increased incidence is likely the result of improved imaging techniques. A recent French prospective study revealed a rate of 13/100, 000/year. Pediatric Stroke is ischemic in 55% and hemorrhagic in 45% (Fig. **1**), while adult stroke is ischemic in up to 85% of patients.

ETIOLOGY

Etiologies in children are diverse and challenging. Cardiac disorders are the commonest predisposition, however, no cause is found in up to 30% of cases. In addition to cardiac-embolic, important causes include genetic, metabolic, degenerative, hematological, vasculitis, infectious, moya moya disease, traumatic, arterial dissection, hypoxic-ischemic encephalopathy, and drugs (cocaine, stimulants, glue stiffing). Inherited genetic and metabolic causes are important in a highly consanguineous population, such as that seen in Saudi Arabia. These etiologies include:

1- Prothrombotic disorders

2- Bleeding disorders

3- Sickle cell disease

4- Inherited cardio-embolic causes

5- Metabolic disorders

6- Degenerative disorders

7- Inherited dyslipidemic states

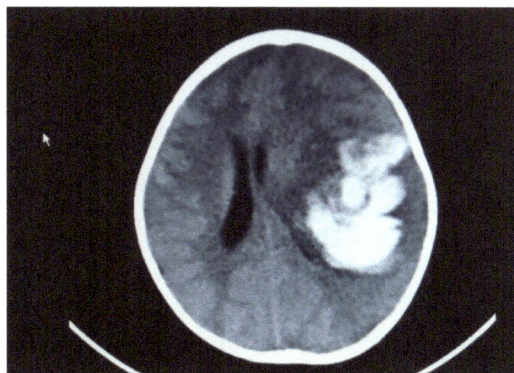

Figure 1: Intracerebral bleeding resulting in acute hemiplegia.

PROTHROMBOTIC DISORDERS

Prothrombotic disorders result in impaired hemostatic system in which the balance is shifted toward thrombosis. These disorders include impairment of vascular endothelium, coagulation cascade, fibrinolytic system, or platelets. In recent studies, up to 50% of thromboembolism is the result of a prothrombotic state. Several prothrombotic disorders were encountered in children with stroke including:

1- Factor V Leiden mutation (commonest)

2- Prothrombin mutation

3- Protein S, C, Antithrombin III deficiency

4- Activated protein C resistance

5- Antiphospholipipid antibodies (lupus anticoagulant, anticardiolipin)

Factor V Leiden (fVL) mutation is the commonest inherited cause of thrombosis. It results from a missense mutation of F5 gene with amino acid substitution making the gene resistant to normal cleavage by activated protein C (APC). Protein C is activated by thrombin and degrades factor Va and VIIIa. The resistance of fVL mutation to APC results in increased thrombin generation and a shift toward increased coagulability. Factor V Leiden mutation affects 5-12% of the general pediatric population. Heterozygous carriers have a 7 fold increased risk of thrombosis, which increases to 80 fold risk for homozygous. The disorder is also associated with adverse maternal and neonatal outcomes including pregnancy related thrombosis, pre-eclampsia, placental abruption and infarction, spontaneous miscarriage, preterm delivery, fetal death, and IUGR. Therefore, history of these disorders is important to be obtained in children with stroke. The mutation was found in up to 21% of hemiplegic cerebral palsy patients compared to 3% of controls. Protein S, C, antithrombin III deficiencies can also be acquired, due to infection, medications (L-asparagenase), hepatic disease, or renal disease. Other blood disorders may predispose to bleeding such as the autosomal recessive Factor I deficiency (congenital afibrinogenemia) and factor VII/VIII deficiency (X linked). Note that intracranial hemorrhage occurs in 2. 6-14% of hemophiliacs and are frequently overlooked. Head injury can be minor; however, the intracranial bleeding is a major cause of death in hemophiliacs.

Suggested coagulation workup in children with stroke

- CBC, PT, PTT

- Plasminogen, Fibrinogen levels

- Protein C, S, Antithrombin II activities

- Activated protein C resistance

- Antiphospholipid Antibodies

- fVL and prothrombin gene mutations

Sickle Cell Disease

Sickle cell disease is a common autosomal recessive hematological disorder that may present with stroke in children, particularly in Saudi Arabia. Stroke occurs in up to 10% with a 50% recurrence risk. It is a more common complication in children less than 10 years of age. The infarction is commonly silent and multiple. Distal occlusive arteriopathy and proximal anterior and middle cerebral artery involvements are characteristic. Transcranial Doppler can help for early detection. Long term hyper-transfusion therapy decreases the recurrence risk to 10% risk; however, allogenic bone marrow transplantation is the treatment of choice.

Metabolic and Degenerative Disorders

A number of metabolic and degenerative disorders may present acutely with hemiplegia including homocystinuria, fabry disease, MELAS, organic acidemias, urea cycle disorders, carbohydrate deficiency glycoprotein syndrome, and menkes disease. Progressive spastic hemiplegia characterize other neurometabolic disorders including juvenile krabbe disease, metachromatic Leukodystrophy, adrenoleukodystrophy, Sturge Weber syndrome, Leigh disease, and subacute sclerosing panencephalitis

MELAS (Mitochondrial Encephalomyopathy, Lactic Acidosis, and Stroke like episodes)

This is a genetic disorder with 25% maternal inheritance. Mothers may be normal or have milder features such as sensory neural deafness or short stature. Four point mutations have been reported in the mitochondrial DNA gene. Symptoms start at 3-35 years of age and in 80% the onset is before 20 years. Recurrent hemiparesis, hemianopsia, cortical blindness, and aphasia may follow a bout of vomiting, headache, abdominal pain, drowsiness, or seizures. The episodes can be spontaneous or triggered by febrile illness. Associated features include retinitis pigmentosa, dementia, hearing loss, and short stature. Serum and CSF lactate are high and brain MRI shows focal leucencies that are bright on T2. These brain lesions are due to a destructive non-ischemic tissue necrosis that is not in a vascular distribution involving both white and grey matter. The parieto-occipital cortex is most frequently involved. Basal ganglia calcification is seen in 30%. Muscle biopsy shows the characteristic ragged red fibers. Mild degree of symptomatic improvement may be seen with treatment with the following vitamin cofactors; coenzyme Q10, phylloquinone, ascorbate, succinate, thiamine, riboflavin, and dichloroacetate (chapter 9).

Familial Hemiplegic Migraine

This is an autosomal dominant disorder (chromosome 19p). Stereotyped events that are frequently triggered by head injury are noted before, during, or after headache. Hemiplegia, hemianesthesia, and aphasia may last for hours to days. They frequently resolve in 2-3 days. The episodes are recurrent and chronic sequlae are rare. Treatment with acetazolamide may provide relief.

Alternating Hemiplegia

This is a rare cause of recurrent hemiplegia in children less than 18 months of age. It is a distinct genetic syndrome linked to migraine resulting from reciprocal translocation 46XY, t3;9(p26;q34). The weakness lasts for minutes to days with associated dystonia, tonic spasms, or episodic nystagmus. The symptoms may disappear with sleep and reappear on awakening. The syndrome is benign, however, chronic sequale have been reported.

Dyslipidemic States

Familial lipid and lipoprotein disorders are rare autosomal dominant defects that result in premature atherosclerotic disease. Most cases have positive family history of early age of onset of ischemic stroke or ischemic heart disease. If suspected, a fasting lipid profile and lipoprotein level should be obtained to document elevated lipoprotein A (LDL like), increased triglecerides, or lowered HDL.

PERINATAL (NEONATAL) STROKE

Perinatal stroke is defined as a cerebrovascular event that occurs between 28 weeks of gestation and 28 days of postnatal age. The incidence, pathogenesis, and clinical features remain poorly categorized. Neonatal stroke comprise up to 25% of pediatric stroke. The suggested prevalence is 24-28/100, 000/year, mostly ischemic in nature. Overall, neonatal stroke is recognized in approximately 1/4000 live births per year. Risk factors include asphyxia (35%), prothrombotic disorders, cardiac disorders, infection, and trauma. However, up to 50% of the cases in full-term neonates were idiopathic. Stroke in the neonatal period is frequently under-recognized clinically. Cases may be asymptomatic for 4-5 months until voluntary hand use develops. However, most neonates present with recurrent seizures during the first 3 days of life. Therefore, only short term treatment with anti-convulsants is recommended. Outcome studies included heterogeneous cohorts including full-term, premature, and asphyxiated neonates with complicated deliveries. The clinical outcome therefore has been very variable. Spastic hemiparesis, recurrent seizures, visual field defect, microcephaly, hypotonia, language, and developmental delay were common; however, many neonates in different series were normal with no residual motor or cognitive deficit. In full term infants with no history of birth asphyxia, the outcome is generally favorable. The likelihood of hemiplegia is higher with abnormal EEG in the first week and/or involvement of internal capsule. The recurrence risk is generally low (3-5%) when compared to 20% in pediatric stroke. Overall, 33% had a normal outcome.

SUMMARY

Although pediatric stroke is uncommon, it should be recognized and investigated promptly. Cardiac disorders are the commonest predisposition, however, no cause is found in up to 30% of cases. In addition to cardiac-embolic, important causes include inherited prothrombotic, genetic, and metabolic disorders, particularly in our community because of the high consanguinity rate. This is an emerging area of clinical research requiring collaborative multidisciplinary effort that includes the neurologist, hematologist, geneticist, and metabolic specialist.

BIBLIOGRAPHY

Jan MM, Camfield PR: Outcome of Neonatal Stroke in Full Term Infants Without Significant Birth Asphyxia. Europ J Ped 1998;157(10):846-848.
Jan MM: Epidemiology of Stroke in Saudi Arabia. Saudi Med J 2001;22:375-6.

CHAPTER 16

Abnormal Movements

Abstract: Movement disorders are relatively common in the pediatric neurology practice. Describing and reading about the characteristics of these movements does not substitute the need to observe them in practice. Once the physician see such movements, recognition becomes easier. All movement disorders are abnormal and involuntary. Most of them disappear in sleep except palatal myoclonus, which is due to a lesion in the central tegmental tract. Identifying abnormal movements depends on their characteristics including whether they are slow or fast, rhythmic or arrhythmic, intermittent or continuous, present at rest or action, and distributed proximally or distally. In this chapter, important movement disorders will be discussed depending on the clinical features rather than the specific disease.

Keywords: Movement disorders, Dyskinesia, Chorea, Athetosis, Tremor, Tics, Dystonia, Myoclonus, Cerebral Palsy, Degenerative, Metabolic.

DYSTONIA

Dystonia is defined as a state of continuous contraction of groups of agonist and antagonist muscles resulting in a sustained abnormal posture, which is frequently twisting in nature. Muscle tone typically fluctuates, varying from normal to extreme hypertonia. Oppenheim first described dystonia in 1911; however, the phenomenology, pathophysiology, and management have become much better understood over the last decade. To organize the clinical and etiologic heterogeneity of dystonia, different classifications have been proposed (Tables 1-3). Clinically, dystonia can be classified according to the age of onset as early (<21 years) or late (>21 years), or according to the distribution of affected body regions as summarized in Table **2**. Dystonic movements usually occur spontaneously. They can be precipitated and/or worsened by attempts to move and can vary with alterations in emotional state and fatigue. However, dystonia typically diminishes or disappears with distraction or sleep. Dystonia can be sub-classified as action induced or posture induced, although secondary dystonia in children is typically present at rest and is increased by action (Table **2**). There are many diverse causes of dystonia. It can be primary (idiopathic) or secondary (symptomatic) to neurodegenerative disorders or other lesions of the brain (Table **1**). However, with the recent mapping of genes for idiopathic dystonias, the term "primary" is becoming outdated. Table **3** summarizes an updated genetic classification and highlights recently mapped genes of various inherited dystonias. Dopa-responsive dystonia is an important cause to recognize because it is treatable. It was first described in 1976 by Segawa. It is a rare inherited primary dystonia plus syndrome (Table **1**). Typically, the patient has a diurnal variation with symptoms that are worse by the end of the day. Dopa-responsive dystonia begins at 1-12 years of age (median 6.5), most often with progressive dystonia in a foot and associated alterations in gait. It should be considered in any child who presents with dystonia of unknown etiology because it responds so dramatically to small doses of L-dopa.

Table 1: Etiologic classification of Childhood Dystonia.

I- Primary (idiopathic)
1-   Primary torsion dystonia (dystonia musculorum deformans)
2-   Segmental (cervical/cranial) dystonia
3-   Sporadic focal dystonia
II- Dystonia plus syndromes
1-   Dystonia with parkinsonism
a-   Dopa-responsive dystonia
b-   Dopamine agonist responsive dystonia
c-   Rapid onset dystonia-parkinsonism
2-   Myoclonus-dystonia syndrome
III- Secondary dystonia
1-   Congenital malformations
2-   Trauma (physical, electric, shock)

Table 1: cont….

3-	Perinatal cerebral injury (anoxia, kernicterus, trauma)
4-	Drug induced (neuroleptics, anticonvulsants, levodopa, cocaine)
5-	Toxic (manganese, cyanide, carbon monoxide, wasp sting)
6-	Infection (encephalitis, HIV, subacute sclerosing panencephalitis)
7-	Endocrine (hypoparathyroidism)
IV- Inherited degenerative disorders	
1-	Autosomal dominant (Juvenile Parkinson's, Huntington's disease)
2-	Autosomal recessive (Wilson's disease, Hallervorden Spatz disease, Neuronal ceroid lipofuscinosis, Gangliosidosis, Lesch Nyhan syndrome, Homocystinuria)
3-	X-linked dominant (Rett syndrome)
4-	X-linked recessive (Dystonia-parkinsonism)
5-	Mitochondrial (Leigh's disease, Leber's disease)
V- Psychogenic dystonia	

Table 2: Clinical classification of Childhood Dystonia.

Classification	Description
A- By distribution	
1- Focal	Eyelids (blepharospasm), mouth (oromandibular dystonia), larynx (spasmodic dysphonia), neck (spasmodic torticollis), hand (writer's cramp)
2- Segmental	
3- Multifocal	Cranial, axial, brachial (arms), or crural (legs)
4- Hemidystonia	Involve 2 or more non-contiguous body parts
5- Generalized	Involve ipsilateral arm and leg
	Both legs plus 1 or more other body part
B- By activation	
1- Task-specific	Only during certain tasks in 1 region (writer's cramp)
2- Action	Only during moving the involved region
3- Overflow	Also induced by moving uninvolved body parts
4- Fixed	Present at rest
5- Paradoxical	Improves by talking or other voluntary movements

Table 3: Updated genetic classification of Dystonia.

Class	Clinical phenotype	Inherit-ance	Locus	Gene
DYT1	Primary torsion dystonia	AD	9q34	Torsin A
DYT2	Primary torsion dystonia	AR	NM	NM
DYT3	Dystonia-parkinsonism	XR	Xq13. 1	NM
DYT4	Whispering dysphonia	AD	NM	NM
DYT5	Dopa-responsive dystonia	AD	14q22. 1	GTPCH-1
		AR	11p15. 5	TH
DYT6	Torsion dystonia, in adults	AD	8p21	NM
DYT7	Familial cervical dystonia	AD	18p	NM
DYT8	Paroxysmal dystonic choreoathetosis	AD	2q33	NM
DYT9	Paroxysmal dyskinesia with spasticity	AD	1p21	NM
DYT10	Paroxysmal kinesigenic dyskinesia	AD	16p11-12	NM
DYT11	Myoclonus-dystonia	AD	7q21	ε-sarcoglycan
DYT12	Dystonia-parkinsonism	AD	19q13	NM
DYT13	Cranial-cervical-brachial	AD	1p36	NM
DYT14	Dopa-responsive dystonia	AD	14q13	NM
DYT15	Myoclonus-dystonia	AD	18p11	NM

NM = Not mapped   **GTPCH-1** = Guanosine-5-triphosphate cyclohydrolase-1   **TH** = Tyrosine hydroxylase

CHOREA

Rapid, jerky, intermittent, random, non-stereotypic, dancing movements that usually affects the proximal extremities and face, but also can involve the distal limbs. They are aggravated by activity and emotional stress, and disappear during sleep. Chorea can be benign (familial or related to exercise or fever). Other causes include cerebral palsy, drugs (antiepileptics, stimulants, and antiemetics), endocrine, collagen vascular (SLE), and genetic disorders (Abetalipoproteinemia, glutaric aciduria, mitochondrial cytopathy, Huntington disease). We frequently encounter mild distal chorea in normal adolescents, particularly girls. Sydenham (rheumatic) chorea is relatively common in developing countries. It can be the only clinical criterion of rheumatic fever and can be unilateral (hemichorea). Ballismus is more violent movements with higher amplitude of flinging choreoform movements. Hemiballismus is the result of a lesion (vascular or neoplastic) in the subthalamic nucleus.

ATHETOSIS

Slow, continuous, writhing movements of the extremities and face, particularly the proximal parts, that is usually combined with chorea (choreoathetosis). They are aggravated by voluntary activity and emotional stimuli. Kernicterus (billirubin encephalopathy) is a usual cause of athetosis without chorea. However, the commonest cause of choreoathetosis remains hypoxic ischemic encephalopathy.

TIC

Tics are complex stereotyped movements that can be incorporated by the child into normal movements. Vocal tics (throat clearing or coughing) can be associated. There is no disruption in the level of consciousness and the movements can be suppressed by the child, however, they are involuntary. Tics increase with stress and never occur in sleep. If tics are due to Tourette syndrome, associated co-morbidities may include attention deficit hyperactivity disorder, obsessive compulsive behaviour, and learning difficulties. Family history of tics or the other co-morbid conditions is frequently positive.

TREMOR

Tremor usually takes the form of rhythmical alternating movements that may occur at rest or action. It can affect the hands, neck, or head (titubation). Action tremor (intention tremor) is aggravated by limb movement. It is a feature of cerebellar disease. Note that the arms have to be adequately stretched during the finger nose test to identify intention tremor as the amplitude of this tremor increases as the finger reaches the target. Resting tremor is relieved by action. It is characteristic of extrapyramidal disorders, such as parkinsonism. Essential (familial) tremor is transmitted in an autosomal dominant pattern. Restlessness or tremulousness is an initial feature followed by the classical action tremor.

Table 4: Etiological classification of Myoclonus.

Etiology	Examples
Physiological	- Anxiety - Exercise - Sleep
Epileptic	- Progressive myoclonic encephalopathies - Neuronal Ceroid Lipofuscinosis - Lafora disease - Mitochondrial encephalopathies
Drugs	- Carbamazepine - Phenytoin - Stimulants - Vigabatrin

Table 4: cont....

Degenerative	- Spinocerebellar degeneration
	- Wilson disease
	- Huntington disease
	- Hallervorden Spatz disease
Metabolic	- Dialysis syndrome
	- Hepatic encephalopathy
	- Renal encephalopathy
Secondary	- Hypoxic ischemic encephalopathy
	- Toxic, Traumatic, Vascular
	- Viral encephalitis

MYOCLONUS

Myoclonus is a sudden, quick, jerky (shock-like) body movement due to contraction of a group of muscles. Myoclonus can be focal (one limb), segmental (palatal, upper or lower limbs), multifocal, or generalized. Palatal myoclonus does not disappear in sleep and usually results from a vascular or neoplastic lesion of the central tegmental tract in the brainstem. Myoclonus can be epileptic or non epileptic. The various causes of myoclonus are summarized in Table **4**. Note that epileptic myoclonus can be drug related in children with severe myoclonic epilepsy of infancy or Lennox Gastaut syndrome. In this situation, myoclonus may appear or is aggravated by carbamazepine, phenytoin, gabapentin, or vigabatrin.

BIBLIOGRAPHY

Jan MM: Misdiagnoses in Children with Dopa-responsive Dystonia. Ped Neurol 2004;31(4):298-303.

CHAPTER 17

Unsteady Gait

Abstract: Unsteady gait and ataxia are relatively common neurological presentation of a variety of acute and chronic disorders. Accurate assessment includes detailed history, examination, and then formulation of a differential diagnosis list to guide laboratory investigations. In this chapter, a clinical approach to the unsteady child is presented with discussion of diagnostic considerations, approach to investigation, treatment, and prognosis.

Keywords: Unsteady, Ataxia, Gait, Paralysis, Weakness, Motor, Sensory, Neuropathy, Myopathy, Cerebellar, Physiotherapy.

INTRODUCTION

Gait unsteadiness is not always due to neurological causes. Simple injuries and musculoskeletal etiologies are most common. It is important to recognize benign and non-neurological causes (Table **1**). Ataxia (lacking order in Greek) refers to a pathologic abnormality of organization or modulation of movement. Although ataxia is most commonly attributable to cerebellar dysfunction, lesions at several levels of the nervous system can result in motor incoordination. Ataxia may be congenital or acquired. Congenital ataxia is usually associated with central nervous system malformations. Acquired ataxia can be classified as acute, chronic, or episodic (Table **2**). Episodic and chronic progressive ataxias are less common in children and are usually caused by inherited metabolic or genetic disorders.

CLINICAL EVALUATION

History

Most children with ataxia are seen because of refusal to walk or abnormal gait (wide-based or drunken gait). Parents less commonly notice the involvement of the arms (tremor), head (titubation), trunk (inability to sit steadily), and speech (dysarthria). At presentation, the primary concern is to exclude serious causes of acute ataxia, including CNS infections and tumors (Table **1**). Detailed history will frequently clarify the cause of the unsteady gait. Inquiry about prior or current symptoms of systemic infection should be included. History of trauma, infection, drug ingestion or headaches may suggest important associations (Table **1**). Recurrent or persistent headache and vomiting or diplopia suggests an intracranial mass lesion and possible elevation of intracranial pressure. A common cause of acute ataxia is inadvertent or deliberate drug ingestion. The child's activities should be reviewed to explore possible exposure to medications, alcohol, and household chemicals. Keep in mind that the causes of acute ataxia are quite different from those of chronic or progressive ataxia. Acute ataxia can be related to trauma, vascular insults, infection, or drug ingestion, while chronic progressive ataxia suggests an inherited metabolic, degenerative, or neoplastic etiology (Table **2**). Recent immunizations should be noted, as should the child's general state of health in the weeks and months prior to presentation. Some inherited metabolic disorders, such as mitochondrial cytopathies and MSUD, may present with intermittent ataxia that resolves slowly (Table **3**). The child may be initially normal in-between the attacks. These episodes are frequently precipitated by infections or drug ingestion (*e.g.* Valproic Acid) and result subsequently in chronic progressive sequale. Accurate past medical and family histories are important in eliciting the possible diagnosis in these situations.

Table 1: Causes of unsteady gait in children.

Foot deformity
Skeletal abnormalities (ankle, knee, or hip joint)
Antalgic gait (due to pain)
Migraine (basilar migraine, benign paroxysmal vertigo)
Raised intracranial pressure (hydrocephalus)
Paretic ataxia (weakness due to upper or lower motor neuron lesion)

Table 1: cont....

Cerebellar Ataxia
Congenital/Genetic
Traumatic (contusion, hemorrhage, post-concussion, vertebral dissection)
Toxic and Drugs (alcohol, antihistamines, anticonvulsants)
Infectious/immune-mediated (chicken pox, ADEM, encephalitis, MS)
Malignancy (medulloblastoma, neuroblastoma)
Paraneoplastic (opsoclonus-myoclonus syndrome)
Vascular (stroke, hypertension, AV malformation, blood disorders)
Degenerative (ataxia telangiectasia)
Post-ictal (epileptic ataxia)
Sensory Ataxia
Guillain-Barré syndrome, chemotherapy, heavy metals, B6, B12 deficiency
Functional Ataxia (including munchausen by proxy syndrome)

ADEM = Acute demyelinating encephalomyelitis   **MS** = Multiple Sclerosis.

Table 2: Types of cerebellar ataxia in childhood.

Acute
Trauma
Toxic and Drugs
Seizure related (post-ictal, nonconvulsive status epilepticus)
Infections/Postinfectious
Vascular (stroke, hypertension, AV malformation, blood disorders)
Malignancy (medulloblastoma, neuroblastoma)
Paraneoplastic (Opsoclonus-myoclonus syndrome)
Functional
Chronic
Congenital (cerebellar hypoplasia, Dandy-Walker and Chiari malformation)
Posttraumatic
Following meningitis/encephalitis
Post-tumor resection or radiation
Hypoxic-ischemic insult
Progressive
Friedreich ataxia
Ataxia Telangiectasia
Sphingolipidosis (gangliosidosis, Niemann-Pick disease)
Leukodystrophies (Pelizaes-Merzbacher, krabbe, metachromatic leukodystrophy)
Mitochondrial disorders (Leigh disease, MERF)
Neuronal ceroid-lipofuscinosis
Progressive myoclonic epilepsies (Lafora disease, Uverricht-Lundborg disease)
Congenital defect of glycosylation
Abetalipoproteinemia
Recurrent
Migraine (basilar migraine, benign paroxysmal vertigo)
Genetic (autosomal dominant episodic ataxias)
Metabolic (amino acidopathies, urea cycle, and mitochondrial disorders)

Table 3: Causes of recurrent intermittent ataxia in childhood.

Migraine and migraine variants
Basilar migraine
Benign paroxysmal vertigo
Benign paroxysmal torticollis of infancy
Alternating hemiplegia of childhood

Table 3: cont….

Genetic disorders
Episodic ataxia type 1 (paroxysmal ataxia with myokymia)
Episodic ataxia type 2 (acetazolamide responsive)
Episodic ataxia types 3 and 4
Episodic ataxia with paroxysmal dystonia
Metabolic disorders
Amino acidopathies
Hartnup disease
Maple syrup urine disease
Urea cycle disorders
Carbamoyl phosphate synthetase deficiency
Ornithine transcarbamylase deficiency
Arginosuccinic aciduria
Organic acidopathies
Biotinidase deficiency
Isovaleric acidemia
Mitochondrial disorders
Pyruvate dehydrogenase deficiency
Leigh disease
Carnitine acetyltransferase deficiency

EXAMINATION

Physical examination can be difficult as ataxic children are often uncooperative and irritable. Observation is needed to look for important signs that may explain the etiology. Look for signs of trauma or meningeal irritation signs. Examination of the eye may provide some clues (*e.g.* conjunctival telangiectasia). Nystagmus is common to disorders affecting the cerebellar hemispheres. Additional abnormalities of cranial nerve examination, such as papilledema and cranial nerve palsies, suggest a space occupying lesion or hydrocephalus. Pupillary abnormalities can be seen with mass lesions, raised intracranial pressure, stroke, or intoxication. Mental status examination in children with postinfectious cerebellar ataxia reveals normal alertness. Abrupt altered responsiveness suggests drug ingestion or toxic exposure.

Extreme irritability can be seen in meningitis, encephalitis, and opsoclonus-myoclonus syndrome. Detailed motor examination is needed to exclude weakness, which may result in hypotonia and incoordination. Cerebellar ataxia is characterized by hypotonia, wide based gait, and dysarthria (fluctuations in clarity, rhythm, tone, and volume). Examination of coordination starts by examining the gait. In cerebellar disease, the patient is off balance with eyes open and worse with eye closure. Walking on a straight line will identify unilateral hemispheric cerebellar disease as the patient will sway towards the affected side. Midline (vermal) lesions cause dysarthria, truncal titubation, and gait abnormalities, whereas lesions of the cerebellar hemispheres spare speech but result in ipsilateral limb hypotonia, dysmetria, and tremor. Tandem walk (walking on a straight line with feet closely attached and alternating in front of each other) is more difficult to perform and may identify subtle cerebellar ataxia. Dysmetria (poor coordination of voluntary movements) results in under or overshooting of limb movements and difficulty with rapid alternating movements (dysdiadochokinesia). Therefore, finger nose or heel shin testing, rapid alternate hand movements or foot tap will test for limb ataxia. Note that the arms have to be adequately stretched during the finger nose test to identify intention tremor as the amplitude of this tremor increases as it reaches the target. The tremor is a to and fro oscillations perpendicular to the approached object. The deep tendon reflexes can be pendular, with slowed contraction and relaxation phases. Detailed sensory examination is needed to exclude sensory ataxia. Particular attention is needed for vibration and position sense examination. Romberg sign will help in testing position sense as the patient stands with outstretched hands and closely placed feet. Off balance with eye closure represents a positive sign, indicating sensory ataxia.

CEREBELLAR ATAXIA

Acute Cerebellar Ataxia

Postinfectious cerebellar ataxia is the most common cause of childhood ataxia, accounting for about 40% of all cases. It usually results from cerebellar demyelination, or less commonly a result of direct cerebellar infection. The demyelination is an autoimmune phenomenon incited by infection or immunization, with subsequent cross-reaction of antibodies against the cerebellum. History of antecedent illness 1-3 weeks before presentation is obtained in about 70% of patients. Numerous infectious agents have been implicated in the pathogenesis of this condition. As many as 26% of cases are preceded by varicella. Rarely, the development of ataxia precedes the eruptive phase of varicella infection. The introduction of universal immunization against varicella is likely to render varicella-related cerebellar ataxia uncommon. The disorder is most common in younger boys (2–4 years) but may be seen in adolescents. Postinfectious cerebellitis presents with the acute gait abnormalities, ranging in severity from unsteadiness and a wide-based stance to complete inability to walk. Symptoms are maximal at onset and may be more severe in cases following varicella infection. The extremities are less affected than the trunk. Acute ataxia is also a common feature of acute demyelinating encephalomyelitis (ADEM), which also develops after a viral illness or vaccination. However, ADEM is distinguished from post-infectious cerebellar ataxia by the occurrence of alteration of consciousness, seizures, and multifocal neurologic deficits. Systemic symptoms such as fever, headache, and meningism are also more common. Repeated episodes of demyelination should raise the concern for multiple sclerosis. Associated findings include optic neuritis and long-tract signs. Head injuries may cause acute ataxia owing to concussion, cerebellar contusion or hemorrhage. After neck injuries, ataxia can point to vertebral artery dissection resulting in ischemic stroke. Cerebellar hemorrhage is rare in childhood and, in the absence of a bleeding diathesis, is most commonly associated with arteriovenous malformations. Acute ataxia is occasionally associated with rapid chaotic multidirectional conjugate eye movements (opsoclonus), myoclonus, and encephalopathy in the so called opsoclonus-myoclonus syndrome. The syndrome can be postinfectious or the presenting manifestation of an occult neuroblastoma. Ataxia in this disorder can be of subacute onset and can fluctuate in association with irritability and recurrent vomiting. Ataxia has also been described as a paraneoplastic phenomenon in other malignancies, such as hodgkin's disease, histiocytosis, and hepatoblastoma. Finally, another important cause of acute ataxia is drug ingestion, including anticonvulsants, benzodiazepines, alcohol, and antihistamines. A high index of suspicion should always be maintained as a history of ingestion or exposure might not be forthcoming. In this situation, the ataxia is often accompanied by mental status changes such as lethargy, confusion, inappropriate speech, or behavior.

Chronic Cerebellar Ataxia

Cerebellar ataxia may result from static (non-progressive) cerebellar anomalies or insults (Table **2**). Congenital causes include cerebellar hemispheric hypoplasia (Fig. **1**), vermal aplasia, basilar impression, and chiari malformation type 1. Cerebellar insults following trauma, infection, hypoxia, or ischemia are usually associated with other motor, developmental and cognitive deficits. In many of these disorders, including cerebral palsy, the child is expected to make some improvements with time. This improvement is not only dependant on the severity of the underlying etiology, but also on associated motor deficits (weakness and spasticity), therapeutic interventions, and rehabilitation.

Progressive Cerebellar Ataxia

Brain tumors are important causes of progressive cerebellar ataxia. Around 50% of all brain tumors arise from the brain stem or cerebellum. Posterior fossa tumors usually present with slowly progressive ataxia and symptoms of increased intracranial pressure. Other clinical features can include headache, papilledema, personality change, and focal neurological abnormalities. Occasionally, supratentorial tumors produce ataxia, usually those in the midline. Parenchymal lesions of the frontal lobes can cause ataxia due to involving frontocerebellar associative fibers. A number of metabolic and degenerative disorders present predominantly with cerebellar ataxia (Table **2**). Progressive ataxia is seen in all patients with ataxia telangiectasia and spinocerebellar ataxias such as Friedreich ataxia. Rare, but treatable disorders should also be considered, such as glucose transporter deficiency syndrome. This disorder is characterized by ataxia, developmental delay, difficult epilepsy, and low CSF glucose (<2. 2 mmol/L). Rapid and impressive improvement is noted after instituting the ketogenic diet.

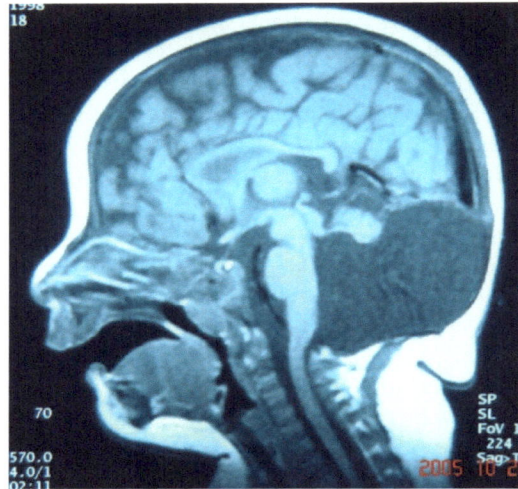

Figure 1: An infant with incoordination and hypotonia due to congenital brain malformation (cerebellar hypoplasia).

Recurrent Cerebellar Ataxia

Occasionally, migraine may present with intermittent ataxia. Less common periodic syndromes of childhood that are precursors to migraine are listed in Table **3**. These syndromes, quite peculiar to children, present a wide variety of episodic symptoms, such as abnormal movements, vomiting, ataxia, and vertigo, and may not include headache at all. Autosomal dominant episodic ataxias are related to mutations in ion channel genes. Treatment with acetazolamide or phenytoin may be helpful. Intermittent ataxia should particularly raise the suspicion of an underlying inborn error of metabolism (Table **3**). Acute exacerbation develops after high protein ingestion, concurrent febrile illness, or other physical stress. This rare presentation occurs mainly in the late infantile and juvenile partial forms of the metabolic disorders listed in Table **3**. Intermittent cerebellar ataxia may or may not be associated with concomitant episodes of stupor and vomiting.

SENSORY ATAXIA

Ataxia can result from loss of sensory input to the cerebellum due to lesions in the posterior column of the spinal cord, roots, or peripheral nerves. Sensory ataxias are characterized by a positive Romberg's sign and decreased deep tendon reflexes. Loss of posterior column sensory functions (proprioception and vibration sense) causes incoordination of the hands and a wide-based, "steppage" gait. These findings worsen with the eyes closed. Sensory ataxia can be seen in children with severe peripheral neuropathy (Dejerine-Sottas disease). Guillain-Barré syndrome (GBS) can result in ataxia, usually in association with weakness and pain. However, ataxia is a rare presenting symptom of GBS. On the other hand, ataxia is characteristic of the less common Miller Fisher variant of GBS, which is a triad of ataxia, areflexia, and ophthalmoplegia. Ataxia is often more marked in the extremities.

INVESTIGATIONS

The primary aim of investigations is to exclude serious conditions, such as brain tumors. A thorough history and physical examination are far more likely to identify the etiology of acute ataxia than is a battery of screening investigations. Of all investigations, drug screen and neuroimaging are most important. However, in the absence of altered consciousness, focal neurologic signs, or marked asymmetry of ataxia, the yield of neuroimaging is low. Acute postinfectious cerebellar ataxia is a diagnosis of exclusion.

Magnetic resonance imaging (MRI) of the brain is normal in most children with postinfectious ataxia. Lesions suggestive of focal cerebellar demyelination are occasionally identified. In ADEM, MRI demonstrates multiple asymmetrically located foci of demyelination within the cerebral and cerebellar white matter. Acute lesions often enhance with gadolinium contrast, reflecting local breakdown of the blood–brain barrier. Neuroimaging is usually normal at presentation of opsoclonus- myoclonus syndrome, however, some degree of cerebellar atrophy can be seen on follow-up imaging. Posterior fossa abnormalities can be difficult to visualize on CT scans, where artifacts sometimes obscure the brain stem and cerebellum. MRI (with diffusion-weighted imaging) is preferred. Cerebrospinal fluid (CSF) examination is commonly normal in postinfectious ataxia and ADEM, with mild pleocytosis and elevation of protein. Mild CSF lymphocytosis provides evidence of an inflammatory process. Significant pleocytosis, low glucose, and elevation of CSF protein suggest meningitis or encephalitis. CSF examination can demonstrate cytoalbuminologic dissociation in more than 90% of patients with GBS. However, the CSF can be normal in the first week of the disease in up to 20% of the patients. Oligoclonal bands and elevation of the serum:CSF immunoglobulin index and myelin basic protein level can be present in post-infectious cerebellar ataxia, ADEM, and MS. Therefore, these findings do not differentiate between the three disorders. Electromyography (EMG) is indicated where sensory ataxia is suspected. In GBS, EMG can be normal at the onset and only shows evidence of proximal demyelination after several days to a week of symptom onset. Urinary excretion of catecholamine metabolites is increased in up to 60% of patients with paraneoplastic opsoclonus-myoclonus syndrome. CT or MRI of the chest and abdomen are needed to identify small tumors. Investigations of children with progressive ataxia are directed towards identifying the underlying etiology and examining associated complications (*e.g.* immune deficiency). The findings on history and physical examination will guide the physician in selecting the required laboratory investigations. For example, if ataxia-telangiectasia is suspected, serum IgA, IgE, and alpha fetoprotein should be obtained. Serum lipid profile is abnormal in abetalipoproteinemia or hypobetalipoproteinemia. Neuroimaging, particularly brain MRI, can show characteristic features in several neurodegenerative disorders such as leukodystrophies and Leigh disease. Frequently, specific diagnostic tests and enzyme assays are needed to reach a definitive diagnosis. These specialized tests are expensive and should be used selectively. They will frequently involve skin fibroblast culture, CSF examination, DNA studies, nerve, or muscle biopsy.

MANAGEMENT

The majority of causes of acute cerebellar ataxia are reversible. In post-infectious cerebellitis, the improvement usually begins after the first week and completes within 3 months. There is no evidence that immunosuppressive therapy, such as steroids, improves the outcome. Recovery from ADEM is typically slower and can be hastened by treatment with corticosteroids. Our protocol involves using 15 mg/kg/day of IV methylprednisolone in four divided doses for 3 days followed by 1 mg/kg/day oral prednisone as single morning dose for 2 weeks. This dose is then tapered slowly over 3-4 weeks. Most patients with ADEM recover completely; however, a minority has significant sequelae. Relapses are rare and should raise the possibility of multiple sclerosis. Brainstem encephalitis should be treated empirically with broadspectrum antibiotics and acyclovir. Treatment of ingestions depends on the nature and amount of the ingested substance. In some cases, administration of an antidote, chelation, dialysis, or other therapies are required. Outcome in most other conditions associated with ataxia is dependent on the underlying disease process. Tumors, stroke, and traumatic brain injury are commonly complicated by significant sequelae. Neuroblastoma should be removed surgically. The underlying tumor is small and well differentiated in most cases of paraneoplastic opsoclonus-myoclonus syndrome. The neurologic syndrome of opsoclonus-myoclonus syndrome can improve slowly; however, most children have long-term neurologic, cognitive and behavioral deficits. Some patients respond to high-dose steroids or intravenous immunoglobulin (IVIG). Children with GBS should be admitted to hospital, with careful monitoring of their respiratory and autonomic function. Specific treatments include IVIG and plasmapheresis. IVIG is safer and should be used when children lose ambulation or develop significant respiratory or bulbar dysfunction. More than 90% of children with GBS recover completely within 3-6 months of disease onset. Chronic ataxia due to static insults and cerebral palsy usually improves with time. Ataxia may persist after operating on children with posterior fossa tumors, particularly in radiated survivors of medulloblastoma.

BIBLIOGRAPHY

Jan MMS: Evaluating the Child with Unsteady Gait. Neurosciences 2009;14(1):3-9.

Jan MMS, Al-Buhairi AR, Baeesa SS: Concise Outline of the Nervous System Examination for the Generalist. Neurosciences 2001;6(1):16-22.

CHAPTER 18

Headache & Migraine

Abstract: Headache is a common complaint, occurring in the majority of school age children. The frequency increases with increasing age and the etiologies range from tension to life-threatening infections and brain tumors. Migraine is the most frequent cause of acute and recurrent headaches in children. Children are usually brought to medical attention to exclude serious causes, such as brain tumors or meningitis. A thorough history, physical and neurological examination, and appropriate diagnostic testing (if indicated) will enable the physician to distinguish tension and migraine headaches from those of a secondary etiology. Children with recurrent headaches are more likely to have certain migraine related phenomena, such as motion sickness, teeth grinding (bruxism), sleep talking and walking (somnambulism), and syncope. Most patients with migraine have type A personality, making them worry allot, perfectionist, and high achievers. This may provide further risks and potential triggers to the recurrent headaches.

Keywords: Headache, Migraine, Aura, Tension, Classic, Common, Confusional, Photophobia, Phonophobia, Brain CT, Pseudotumor.

EPIDEMIOLOGY

More than 90% of school age children suffer from headaches. Overall, the prevalence of non-migraine headaches is 10-25%. In the acute setting (emergency room), many children with acute headache have a viral illness or an upper respiratory infection (*e.g.* sinusitis, otitis media). In the outpatient department, psychosocial (*e.g.* family or school problems) and infectious etiologies are common. Tension-type headache (TTH) and migraine are the two most common types in children and adolescents. Migraine constituted up to 75% of referrals for childhood headache in one series. The prevalence of migraine headaches is 4-5% among 3-11 years old children with an increasing prevalence with age. The female-to-male ratio also changes with age. The prevalence is greater in boys before age seven years, is equivalent in boys and girls between ages 7 and 11 years, and is greater in adult women than in men (ratio 3:1).

PATHOPHYSIOLOGY

Muscles attached to the skull are the possible source of pain in TTH; however, the pathophysiology is largely unknown. The smaller genetic effect on TTH than on migraine suggests that the two disorders are distinct. However, many believe that TTH and migraine represent the same pathophysiological spectrum. The old belief that the migraine aura is due to cerebral vasoconstriction and the headache is due to vasodilatation has been abandoned. Recent evidence suggests spreading cortical depression during the aura and neurogenic inflammation, due to increased cellular permeability, causing the pulsatile headache. Note that the brain itself is painless. Vascular instability in the pain sensitive structures (dura, larger vessels, roots, and nerves) is responsible for the headache while the aura is a cortical phenomenon. Increased intracranial pressure causes pain mainly by the traction and displacement of intracranial arteries.

CLINICAL EVALUATION

Headache may not be apparent to parents of younger children who may present with excessive crying, colic, rocking, or hiding. Chronic headache may result in developmental regression, social withdrawal, and behavior problems. Older children are better able to perceive, localize, and remember pain. Emotional, behavioral, and personality factors become more important as the child enters adolescence. The history of headache provides most of the necessary diagnostic information in the evaluation of childhood headaches (Table **1**). A thorough history helps to focus the physical examination and prevent unnecessary investigations and neuroimaging. The history of headache should be obtained from both parents and the child, who may add valuable diagnostic information (*e.g.* visual migraine aura). The following history details should be obtained including age of onset, precipitating and relieving factors, aura, time and mode of onset, location, frequency, severity (effect on activity and school attendance), quality (throbbing or pulsatile in migraine), duration, associated symptoms (photophobia, phonophobia, nausea, vomiting), effect of physical activity (migraine increases with exercise), and response to treatment. A diary, in which the quality, location, severity, timing, precipitating factors, and associated features of the headache are recorded prospectively, is a useful adjunct. A diary is not subject to recall error, may reveal a pattern that is typical for a certain type of headache, and provides important diagnostic information for children who are unable to provide sufficient detail during the clinic visit. In acute headaches, questions concerning symptoms of increased intracranial pressure are particularly important (Table 2). The presence of these features is an indication for further evaluation and/or neuroimaging. The following features are suggestive of raised intracranial pressure including sleep-related or early morning headache (intracranial pressure is higher during lying down), persistently localized headache of recent onset, progressive increase in headache frequency or severity, personality change, persistent vomiting without nausea, and headache worsened by cough, micturation, or defecation. In chronic headaches, it is important to appreciate the potential co-existence of other chronic disorders, such as asthma or diabetes. Headache also can be a side effect of many medications including bronchodilators, stimulants, and some antiepileptic drugs (*e.g.* lamotrigine). Family history of headache or migraine, particularly maternal, is commonly encountered in children with migraine.

Table 1: The international classification of headache disorders II.

Tension-type headache (TTH)	
A	At least 10 episodes fulfilling B-D criteria
	Episodic or Chronic (lasting for >15 days)
B	30 min - 7 days in duration
C	At least 2 of the following four criteria:
	1- Non-pulsating (pressing or tightening)
	2- Mild to moderate
	3- Bilateral
	4- Not increased by exercise
D	Both of the following:
	1- No nausea or vomiting
	2- No photophobia or phonophobia, or 1 but not both
E	Not attributed to another disorder
Migraine without aura	
A	At least 5 attacks fulfilling B-D criteria
B	4-72 hr in duration
C	At least 2 of the following four criteria:
	1- Unilateral
	2- Pulsatile
	3- Moderate to severe
	4- Increase by exercise
D	At least 1 of the following two criteria:
	1- Nausea and/or vomiting
	2- Photophobia and phonophobia
E	Not attributed to another disorder
Migraine with aura	
A	At least 2 attacks fulfilling B-D criteria
B	Aura of 1 of the following criteria, but no motor weakness:
	1- Reversible positive or negative visual features
	2- Reversible positive or negative sensory features
	3- Reversible dysphasic speech disturbance
C	At least 2 of the following criteria:
	1- Homonymous visual and/or unilateral sensory symptoms
	2- Aura symptoms develops gradually over ≥5min
	3- Aura 5-60min in duration
D	Migraine without aura begins during the aura or within 60min
E	Not attributed to another disorder

Table 2: Important symptoms and signs that may suggest raised intracranial pressure or a space occupying lesion (Red Flags).

SYMPTOMS	
1-	New onset headache
2-	Headache persistent in one site
3-	Headache progressive in severity or frequency
4-	No relief with regular analgesics
5-	Sleep-related or early morning headache
6-	Worsened by cough, micturition, or defecation
7-	Persistent vomiting without nausea
8-	Personality change
9-	Other neurological symptoms (seizures, double vision, weakness)
SIGNS	
1-	Macrocephaly
2-	Bulging anterior fontanel
3-	Lethargy
4-	Neck stiffness
5-	Neurocutaneous signs
6-	Papilledema
7-	Focal neurological signs (motor, sensory, cerebellar)

INTERNATIONAL CLASSIFICATION OF HEADACHES

The recently developed International Classification of Headache Disorders, second edition (ICHD-II) was the result of many years' work by many headache experts from different countries. ICDH-II criteria are superior to the earlier ICDH-I and International Headache Society (IHS) criteria in identifying definite migraine in children and adolescents. These diagnostic criteria are summarized in Table **1**. The terms "common" and "classic" migraine are no longer used. Differentiating the first migraine episode from symptomatic headache (*e.g.* caused by infection or neoplasm) may be difficult because the diagnostic criteria would not have been met. Simpler and easier diagnostic criteria were developed earlier by Prensky. It requires recurrent headaches separated by symptom-free intervals and at least three of the following six symptoms or criteria: 1) abdominal pain, nausea or vomiting, 2) localized unilateral or hemicranial headaches, 3) throbbing, pulsatile quality to the pain, 4) complete relief after a brief period of sleep, 5) visual or sensory aura, and 6) family history of migraine. The Prensy criteria are applicable to children and can be used in the clinic as an initial screen. The ICHD-II is useful for more accurate case definitions and reporting in clinical research. However, some authors suggested that these criteria may be too restrictive to differentiate TTH from migraine without aura in children.

TENSION-TYPE HEADACHES

Tension-type headache (TTH) is characterized by bilateral pressing or constricting tightness that occurs anywhere on the head (Table **1**). The headache is non-throbbing, is of mild to moderate intensity, and lasts from 30 minutes to several days, *i.e.* can be prolonged. The patient may have increased tenderness on pericranial manual palpation. TTH is not accompanied by nausea or vomiting nor aggravated by routine physical activities, which are migraine features. Stress (good or bad) is the usual trigger. Sometimes, the overlap of some of the symptoms of migraine can make the differentiation difficult. As well, the co-occurrence of migraine and TTH is frequent, *i.e.* many patients have more that one headache type.

MIGRAINE HEADACHE

Migraine is characterized by recurrent episodes of headache that are aggravated by exercise and relieved by sleep (Table **1**). Autonomic symptoms are commonly seen and include photophobia, phonophobia, nausea, and vomiting. Reversible aura can take several forms including visual features that can be positive (*e.g.*

flickering lights, spots, lines) or negative (vision loss, homonymous field defect), sensory features that also can be positive (*e.g.* pins and needles) or negative (numbness), or dysphasic speech disturbance (Table **1**). The aura typically develops gradually over 5 minutes and lasts for less than one hour. The headache may occur during or within 60 minutes of the aura symptoms. Occasionally, migraine aura occurs without headache (acephalgic migraine). Compared to adults, migraine in children is more likely to be bilateral (bifrontal or bitemporal) with shorter duration. Migraine in infants and toddlers may be more difficult to recognize, with symptoms of head holding, irritability, vomiting, pallor, and head tilt, all relieved by sleep. Hemicrania continua is a rare neurological emergency with continuous unilateral headache that usually responds to indomethacin.

MIGRAINE VARIANTS

The migraine variants are unique to pediatrics and are a fascinating and challenging group of disorders characterized by several clinical and neurological features. Migraine may be complicated by ophthalmoplegia, recurrent vomiting, hemiplegia, ataxia, and confusion (Table **3**). These unusual features are associated with recurrent migraine headaches and family history of migraine. However, all the variants discussed in Table **3** represent diagnoses of exclusion. Therefore, these children should be thoroughly evaluated by careful medical history, physical examination, and appropriate neurodiagnostic studies, to exclude other diagnoses (*e.g.* intracranial tumor, hemorrhage, or infection). Often, these unusual features initially lead the clinician in the direction of epilepsy, cerebrovascular, traumatic, or metabolic disorders. Only after detailed evaluation does the diagnosis become apparent. Recognition of the typical feature may help in preventing unnecessary investigations and hospital admission of some of these children.

Table 3: Important migraine variants.

Visual
- Opthalmoplegic migraine
- Retinal migraine
- Transient post-traumatic cortical blindness
Gastrointestinal
- Cyclic vomiting
- Recurrent vomiting following minor head injury
- Infant colic
Motor
- Paroxysmal torticollis
- Hemiplegic migraine
- Benign paroxysmal vertigo
- Basilar Migraine
Psychic
- Acute confusional migraine
- Alice in wonderland phenomenon

1- Migraine Variants with Visual Features

The visual aura associated with migraine has been discussed earlier in the migraine headache section. Several other visual variants can be associated with migraine including opthalmoplegic migraine, retinal migraine, and transient post-traumatic cortical blindness. In ophthalmoplegic migraine, ipsilateral oculomotor palsy may last for up to 4 weeks. Retinal migraine is rare in children and manifests by attacks of transient monocular vision loss associated with migraine headaches. Vision loss usually lasts less than 1 hour; however, irreversible defects may occur with recurrent attacks representing migrainous retinal infarction. Transient cortical blindness is characterized by normal pupillary response and fundoscopy, and follows minor head trauma. Associate migraine symptoms occur with vision returning to normal within minutes to hours after the trauma leaving no neurological sequelae.

2- Migraine Variants with Gastrointestinal Features

The so called "abdominal migraine" is no longer recognized as a migraine variant in the latest ICHD-II guidelines. An organic pathology is more likely responsible for symptoms of episodic abdominal pain with nausea and vomiting that are not associated with headaches. Recognized migraine variants with prominent gastrointestinal symptoms include cyclic vomiting, recurrent vomiting following minor head injury, and infant colic (Table **3**). Jan et al found migraine headaches, motion sickness, and family history of migraine highly predictive of recurrent vomiting after minor head injury. Recognition of this association will reduce extensive investigations and hospitalization of selected children with minor trauma and no focal neurological features. We also found a strong association between migraine headaches and history of infantile colic. The pain and crying in some of these genetically predisposed infants could represent a form of migraine with an age specific clinical expression. Favorable response to anti-migraine treatment is also supportive; however, such diagnosis should be made after careful exclusion of organic causes of infant colic, such as milk allergy, otitis media, urinary tract infection, intestinal obstruction, and hypertension.

3- Migraine Variants with Motor Features

Benign paroxysmal torticollis, comprised of recurrent, often short-lived, and spontaneously recovering attacks of head tilt in infants, also has been proposed as a migraine variant. Migraine can also be complicated with hemiplegia (hemiplegic migraine), which can lead erroneously to the diagnosis of stroke. The diagnosis is by exclusion. Familial alternating hemiplegia has been also linked to migraine. Such diagnoses should be made only after excluding cerebrovascular disorders.

4- Migraine Variants with Psychic Features

Sudden state of confusion and agitation with migraine characterize acute confusional migraine. The episode can follow mild head injury and is more common in boys. Alice in wonderland phenomenon is an interesting syndrome manifesting with recurrent episodes of impaired time sense, body image, and visual analysis of the environment. The child would report that objects and people look smaller or larger, closer or farther, and slower or faster than normal. The symptoms occur with a clear state of consciousness and in the absence of any evidence of an encephalitic process, seizures, drug ingestion, or psychiatric illness.

PHYSICAL EXAMINATION

The physical examination often is normal in children with tension or migraine headaches. Normal blood pressure should be documented. Measurement of height, weight, and head circumference, auscultation of the head for bruit (a sign of arteriovenous malformation) are important aspects of the examination. Detailed neurological examination is needed to exclude focal neurological signs. Lethargy, macrocephaly, focal neurological signs, neck stiffness, neurocutaneous signs, or papilledema should raise the suspicion of a space-occupying lesion (Table **2**). However, note that most brain tumors in childhood are midline (*e.g.* medulloblastoma, cerebellar astrocytoma, and craniopharyngioma) with minimal lateralizing physical findings. Papilledema may be difficult to appreciate in the young or uncooperative child and therefore ophthalmologic assessment is needed.

LABORATORY EVALUATION

Laboratory testing is rarely helpful in the evaluation of childhood headache. Lumbar puncture (LP) is necessary if intracranial infection or pseudotumor cerebri are suspected clinically. Neuroimaging typically is performed before LP because LP is contraindicated in patients with space-occupying lesions. However, in patients with suspected bacterial meningitis, the risks of delaying the LP and administration of antibiotics while awaiting neuroimaging must be considered. Patients in whom pseudotumor cerebri is suspected may require reassurance or sedation before undergoing the lumbar puncture because an accurate opening pressure measurement is crucial for accurate diagnosis. Electroencephalography (EEG) is not useful in evaluating children with headaches unless epilepsy is suspected.

NEUROIMAGING

Children who have signs or symptoms of an intracranial process should undergo urgent neuroimaging with computed tomography (CT) or Magnetic resonance Imaging (MRI) (Table **2**). These studies may detect a variety of disorders that cause headache, including trauma, infections, neoplasms, or vascular disorders. CT typically is performed in acute situations in which hemorrhage is suspected or rapid diagnosis of a space-occupying lesion is necessary. MRI usually is preferred in other situations, or if there is persistent concern despite a normal CT scan. MRI demonstrates sellar lesions, craniocervical junction lesions, white matter abnormalities, and congenital anomalies more accurately than does CT. However, MRI may require heavy sedation and is more expensive and time-consuming than is CT. Magnetic resonance venography (MRV) is recommended for children with pseudotumor cerebri to exclude venous sinus abnormalities, including thrombosis. Most patients with migraine headaches do not need neuroimaging; nor do children who have chronic non-progressive headaches with no signs or symptoms of increased intracranial pressure. Studies have documented that all of the children with surgically treatable lesions had abnormal findings on neurological examination, including papilledema, abnormal eye movements, and motor or gait dysfunction. The Quality Standards Subcommittee of the American Academy of Neurology and the Practice Committee of Child Neurology Society recommendations for neuroimaging of children and adolescents with recurrent headaches unassociated with trauma, fever, or other obvious provocative cause, concluded that routine neuroimaging is not indicated if the neurological examination is normal. Neuroimaging should be considered in children with recent onset of severe headache, change in the headache type, associated focal neurological features, or seizures.

MANAGEMENT

An important step in the management is to exclude serious intracranial pathology and reassure the child and the parents. This by itself may alleviate associated anxieties and result in reduction of the headache severity and frequency. We always advice the older children or the parents of younger children to document in a diary the headache occasions and associated activities and symptoms in the preceding 24 hours. This would help in identifying the triggers and therefore trying to avoid them. Simple analgesics in appropriate doses are usually effective at the beginning of the headache. Typically, acetaminophen (Panadol or Tylenol) is used at 20 mg/kg/dose. A common pitfall is to use subtherapeutic doses or use the analgesic late, after the symptoms became severe and therefore less responsive to simple analgesics. If not effective, stronger nonsteroidal analgesics (*e.g.* Ibuprofen) or abortive therapy (Triptans) can be used. Narcotics should be avoided because of the risk of dependency. Chronic daily headaches (CDH) are often linked to abuse of pain medications. Therefore, the physician should enquire about the dose and frequency of pain medications in every patient. Treatment of CDH includes neck physiotherapy for stiffness, withdrawal of the abused drug, and treatment of any withdrawal symptoms. Recurrent headaches unresponsive to standard therapy or resulting in significant social limitations or absence from school can be treated prophylactically for 3-6 months. Drugs that can be used ordered in our preference include Cyproheptidine (Periactin), Valproic Acid, Topiramate, or Gabapentin. The parents should understand that these drugs are not analgesics and that they should be taken regularly to decrease headache recurrences. Recently, relaxation exercises (self hypnosis) were found very effective in aborting the headaches in older children and adolescents.

BIBLIOGRAPHY

Jan MMS: Updated Overview of Pediatric Headache and Migraine. Saudi Med J 2007;28(9):1324-9.

Jan MMS, Camfield PR, Gordon K, Camfield CS: Vomiting After Mild Head Injury Is Related To Migraine. J Pediatr 1997;130:134-7.

Jan MMS: History of Motion Sickness Is Predictive of Childhood Migraine. J Paediatr Child Health 1998;34(5):483-484.

Jan MMS: Criteria for Diagnosing Migraine and Tension Headaches. Saudi Med J 1999;20(4):325-326.

Jan MMS, Al-Buhairi AR: Is Infantile Colic A Migraine Related Phenomenon? Clin Pediatr 2001;40:295-297.

CHAPTER 19

Demyelinating Disorders

Abstract: Two important acute demyelinating disorders will be discussed in this chapter; multiple sclerosis (MS) and acute disseminated encephalomyelitis (ADEM). The distinction between the two disorders can be problematic, but in this chapter, a concise summary of these two disorders will be presented. Childhood MS is rare and has different genetic risk factors and similar clinical and MRI findings to adult onset MS. Exposure to extrinsic environmental factors during early childhood in genetically predisposed individuals is believed to trigger MS.

Keywords: Multiple sclerosis, Ataxia, Gait, Paralysis, Weakness, Motor, Sensory, White matter, Myelopathy, Cerebellar, Demyelination.

CHILDHOOD MULTIPLE SCLEROSIS

Onset of MS is extremely uncommon in early childhood, particularly in those less than 10 years of age. However, childhood MS is being increasingly recognized. The increased awareness may be the result of early recognition or genuine increase in the proportion of MS patients presenting during childhood. Despite this, there are several barriers to early diagnosis as many physicians still view MS as an exclusively adult disease and therefore, may not consider the diagnosis in children. As well, both clinical and radiological diagnostic criteria have not been validated in children.

EPIDEMIOLOGY

MS is rare in children; however, the exact prevalence is unknown. At least 5% of all MS patients have their first attack before 16 years of age. The overall prevalence varies significantly from 1-10/100, 000 people in Japan to 248/100, 000 in Canada. Regions further from the equator (Canada and north Europe) are high risk regions; however, MS does occur in all studied populations. The point prevalence of MS in a regional population of Saudi Arabia has been estimated at 0.04. Epidemiological studies have shown that individuals who migrate during childhood to high risk areas adopt the MS risk of their new country rather than maintaining the MS risk of their original country. Although environmental exposures may play a role, genetic influences are also contributory. Specific human leukocyte antigens (HLA) have been associated with increased MS risk in certain populations. MS patients are more likely to carry HLA DRB1, DQA1, and DQB1 loci. As well, patients with HLA-DR15 had an earlier onset of their disease. MS susceptibility in these people interacts with many other factors including immunologic, environmental, and myelin-related genes. Familial cases of MS have been well documented. The risk of MS in first degree relatives is about 5% compared to the 0.2% risk in the general population with a 30% concordance in identical twins. Individual risk of MS increases with the number of affected relatives and with their earlier age of onset. The female to male ratio of adult MS is 2.5:1. In contrast, the female to male ratio in children is 1.4:1. The lower female predominance in children suggests a hormonal factor in pathophysiology.

CLINICAL MANIFESTATIONS

Overall, childhood MS most commonly present in adolescence. In a study of 149 children younger than 16 years presenting with MS, 73% presented with an initial attack after 13 years of age. MS is characterized by multiple episodes of neurological dysfunction secondary to inflammatory CNS demyelination. The most characteristic presentation includes sensory, motor, and brainstem signs and symptoms. Involvement of the pyramidal system is the most common mode of presentation in young Saudi patients. Episodes must be due to different CNS involvements (optic nerve, brain, spinal cord) and separated by more than 30 days interval. Approximately 90% of children with MS present with this relapsing-remitting pattern, which is similar to adult MS. Relapses occur in the first 2 years in the majority of cases; however, up to 14% of children with MS had the second attack more than 10 years after the initial presentation. Primary progressive MS, characterized by worsening neurological disability over time in the absence of clear attacks, is extremely uncommon in children. The clinical features of MS reflect the site of active CNS demyelination. Optic neuritis is a common initial manifestation that is characterized by progressive visual loss with decreased color perception and associated pain on eye movements. When compared to adults, optic neuritis in children is often bilateral. At initial presentation, optic neuritis is associated with an increased risk of subsequent MS. In a long term follow up study, 26% were ultimately diagnosed with MS, sometimes many years after the initial episode of optic neuritis. Younger children (less than 6 years) commonly present with ataxia or seizures. A rare MS variant is Devic's syndrome (neuromyelitis optica), which is characterized by acute transverse myelitis and bilateral optic neuritis. The clinical outcome of Devic's syndrome is generally poor.

INVESTIGATIONS

No single laboratory finding is necessary or sufficient for diagnosing MS. CSF fluid analysis often shows pleocytosis (66%), increased oligoclonal bands and intrathecal IgG synthesis. Increased oligoclonal bands are used in conjunction with serial MRI findings to confirm the diagnosis of MS. Oligoclonal bands in the CSF were present in 75% of children with clinically definite MS. The percentage increases to 81% with the advance of the disease. Recently, isoelectric focusing was found to be superior to the traditional agarose gel electrophoresis in detecting oligoclonal bands in the CSF with a sensitivity of 91% and a specificity of 96% in adult MS patients. CSF examination is also useful to exclude CNS infection or malignancy. MRI features typically include multiple lesions in the periventricular, subcortical, infratentorial, and spinal cord white matter as shown in Fig. **1**.

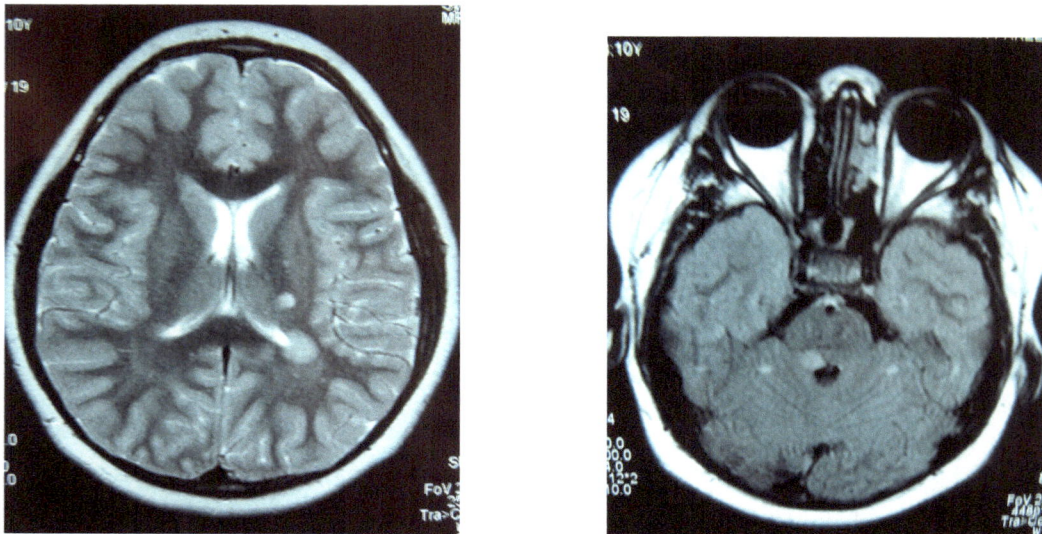

Figure 1: MRI in a child with multiple sclerosis showing multiple periventricular (top) and brain stem (bottom) hyperintense patches.

Cortical gray matter lesions are either not present or rare. Serial MR Images revealing new gadolinium-enhancing lesions, or new lesions on T2-weighted images, can be used to document progressive disease activity even in the absence of new clinical symptoms and signs. Pediatric MS patients are less likely to meet the diagnostic MRI criteria when compared to adults. In fact, many experts believe that childhood MS is a clinical diagnosis, particularly that some children with definite MS may not meet all MRI criteria. Occasionally, neuroimaging reveals atypical large or nodular demyelinating lesions that can be mistaken for tumors. It is important to consider MS in these children in order to avoid unnecessary neurosurgical interventions. MS activity can be evaluated by using evoked potentials. Prolonged or absent visual and somatosensory evoked potentials can provide evidence of additional lesions in the optic pathway or spinal cord.

DIFFERENTIAL DIAGNOSES OF MS

Because MS is rare in children, several other causes of acquired demyelination should be considered. The most important differential diagnosis at initial presentation is acute disseminated encephalomyelitis (ADEM). The differentiating clinical, laboratory, and radiological features of ADEM and MS are summarized in Table **1** and discussed further in the next section. However, the distinction in practice can be difficult, particularly at initial presentation. As well, multiphasic ADEM has been described with recurrent symptoms 3-6 years after initial presentation. Other differential diagnoses include infectious causes (Lyme disease, syphilis, HIV, Brucellosis), CNS vasculitis such as systemic lupus erythematosus (SLE), CNS lymphoma, and neurosarcoidosis. Leukodystrophies and mitochondrial encephalopathy can be easily differentiated based on the clinical and radiological data. Several investigations can help in excluding other etiologies including brain MRI, serum and CSF viral studies, Lyme disease serology, serum lactate, serum markers for SLE (antinuclear antibody, double-stranded DNA). Further detailed tests are not indicated routinely and should be individualized and based on the clinical and radiological findings.

Table 1: Differentiating clinical, laboratory and MRI features.

Feature	ADEM	MS
History of recent infection or vaccination	Common	Rare
Systemic symptoms	Common	Rare
Fever	43%	6%
Headache	57%	24%
Fatigue	71%	29%
Vomiting	57%	0%
Encephalopathy	71%	6%
Seizures	Common	Rare
Isolated optic neuritis	Less common (23%)	Common
Severity of illness	Usually severe	Less severe
CSF oligoclonal bands	29%	75%
MRI changes		
Periventricular distribution	50%	91%
Corpus callosum lesions	17%	64%
Recurrence	Rare	Common

ADEM = Acute disseminated encephalomyelitis   **MS** = Multiple sclerosis

ACUTE DISSEMINATED ENCEPHALOMYELITIS

ADEM is an uncommon autoimmune inflammatory demyelinating disease. The mechanism proposed is that myelin autoantigens share antigenic determinants with those of an infecting pathogen. Antiviral antibodies or a cell mediated response to the pathogen cross react with the myelin autoantigens, resulting in ADEM. ADEM usually follows an infection of the upper respiratory tract or immunization. The clinical features include fever or other systemic signs such as nausea, vomiting, headache, irritability, and neck stiffness. The neurological signs are variable and depend upon the location of the CNS involvement. The disease is usually diffuse, and children often present with multifocal signs. The most common neurological signs were motor deficits (*e.g.* ataxia, hemiparesis) and impaired consciousness. Cranial nerve abnormalities, including optic neuritis with vision impairment, gaze paresis, facial weakness, and swallowing difficulties, occurred frequently. Progression of neurological signs to the maximum deficit occurred over one week on average. ADEM typically lasts from two to four weeks. Development of signs can be more gradual, lasting up to one month, or occur acutely with rapid progression. Treatment of ADEM is similar to an acute MS attack (see next section). Patients with ADEM usually recover slowly, over four to six weeks. Children usually recover completely, although some have neurological sequelae. ADEM is considered a monophasic illness. Patients who appear to have an early relapse may in fact have a protracted clinical course or treatment failure, rather than a new episode. Relapse after a few months suggest the possibility of multiphasic disseminated encephalomyelitis. If relapse occurs after six months or there is progressive neurological deterioration, the diagnosis of MS should be considered.

MANAGEMENT

The psychological impact of MS on the child and adolescent may also be profound. Psychological advice and support is needed for many of these children and their families. Studies in adults suggest that early treatment may prevent or delay the occurrence of clinically definite MS and that disease modifying drugs can reduce the burden of the disease. Intravenous (IV) methylprednisolone speeds recovery from an acute MS relapse. In optic neuritis, IV steroids resulted in rapid recovery of vision and delay in the subsequent diagnosis of MS. Acute MS exacerbations in our pediatric MS patients are treated with 15 mg/kg/day of IV methylprednisolone in four divided doses for 3 days followed by 1 mg/kg/day oral prednisone as single morning dose for 2 weeks. This dose is then tapered slowly over 3-4 weeks. Other institutions may use higher doses reaching 30 mg/kg once daily without maintenance doses. Some children do not respond to steroids or develop recurrent symptoms during the prednisone taper. These children are treated with 1 g/kg/day IV immunoglobulin (IVIG) for two days. Monthly IVIG is required for 3-6 months in some children to improve clinical symptoms or to allow withdrawal of steroid therapy.

Several other immunomodulatory (disease-modifying) therapies have been used in MS. Interferon-β (Rebif) and interferon-β 1a (Avonex) have been shown to reduce the frequency of clinical relapses by 30% in patients with relapsing remitting MS. Interferon therapy has been also shown to reduce the progression of disability and inflammatory activity as assessed by gadolinium enhancement on MRI. This favorable response has been also documented in an open label study from Saudi Arabia. There is increasing evidence supporting the impact of early therapy on long-term physical and cognitive outcome of adult MS. However, there are limited reports on the use of interferons in children. Liver function tests and complete blood count studies should be monitored every 3 months. Transaminase elevation necessitates reduction in the dose. Flu-like side effects have been noted in 20% of children on interferons, which is usually managed easily with analgesics. Although interferons were well tolerated, prospective randomized studies are needed to determine if there is long term benefit in the pediatric population. Finally, cyclophosphamide has been used in MS with variable success. Careful review of the literature suggests that cyclophosphamide may be helpful in children with frequent relapses or very aggressive MS that failed other treatments. Potential risks of this therapy include immunosuppression, malignancy, and infertility.

PROGNOSIS

Childhood MS appears to be less severe than the adult form. However, this is not a universal finding and severe disability can occur with childhood MS, particularly in younger children. The presence of seizures seems to carry a poor prognosis in terms of death or primary progressive course. Children with this chronic disease are at increased risk of experiencing chronic fatigue, emotional, cognitive, and school difficulties. Adolescents with MS frequently report difficulty with higher cortical functions and multiple task organization. Cognitive deficits may occur early in as many as 65% of patients. Children are at higher risk because of the impact on ongoing development and maturation. In addition to cognitive decline, motor and visual disabilities are the most commonly encountered. Over time, approximately 70% of relapsing remitting MS patients will experience progressive motor disability in the absence of a definable attack (secondary progressive MS). The time from initial presentation to this advanced stage is 10-15 years in 50% of MS patients. However, the disease progression and disability scores are generally less severe in childhood MS, with 76% of patients still ambulating 15 years after initial diagnosis.

SUMMARY

MS is rare in children and the etiology remains unknown. Research into the earliest events in MS pathogenesis is needed to enhance our information of this disease. As well, understanding the triggers and initial immunologic targets involved may lead to the development of new therapies. Both clinical research and patient management will be enhanced by clinical and MRI criteria validated in the pediatric MS population and by increased knowledge of the safety and efficacy of immunomodulatory therapies. Prospective longitudinal studies are required to evaluate the physical, cognitive, and psychosocial impact of childhood MS and the long term benefit of various therapeutic modalities.

BIBLIOGRAPHY

Jan MMS. Childhood Multiple Sclerosis. J Pediatr Neurol 2005;3(3):131-6.

CHAPTER 20

DNR Decisions

Abstract: Cardiopulmonary resuscitation (CPR) is now routinely performed on any hospitalized patients who suffer cardiac or respiratory arrest. Children with irreversible or progressive terminal illness may benefit temporarily from CPR, only to deteriorate later on. Painful and invasive procedures may be performed unnecessarily and the child could be left in a worse condition. A "do not resuscitate" (DNR) order indicates that the treating team has decided not to have CPR attempted in the event of cardiac or pulmonary arrest. In this chapter, various aspects related to the DNR decision making in children will be discussed and summary of the published guidelines by the Royal College of Pediatrics & Child Health and the American Academy of Pediatrics will be presented.

Keywords: DNR, Resusitation, Brain death, EEG, Isotope scan, Conciousness, Unresponsiveness, Vegetative, MRI, Ventillation.

BACKGROUND

Both pediatricians and parents have the common purpose of restoring health and sustaining the life of the child. Medical advances make it possible to achieve this objective in circumstances previously regarded as hopeless. This capability brings with it considerable clinical, moral, socio-cultural, legal and economic issues that challenge the values and goals of pediatric care. While these issues arise in many settings, they are most evident in the pediatric intensive care units (PICU). Cardiopulmonary resuscitation (CPR) is now routinely performed on any hospitalized patients who suffer cardiac or respiratory arrest. Consent to administer CPR is presumed because of the urgency of a life threatening situation and since the family decisions may be clouded during such acute situations. The frequent performance of CPR on patients who are terminally ill or who have little chance of surviving has prompted concern that resuscitation efforts may be employed too broadly. Advanced invasive procedures and treatments that may promote and sustain life may not confer any foreseeable benefit and in fact may cause further suffering to the child and the family. Therefore, CPR may be withheld if, in the judgment of the treating team, an attempt to resuscitate the patient would be futile. However, the practical decision of "do not resuscitate" (DNR) is always difficult and should signal a change in focus towards palliative care. It is important to make sure that the child is as comfortable as possible and in no circumstances is it appropriate to withhold such palliative care.

ETHICAL ISSUES

When DNR is considered, four fundamental ethical principles apply as shown in Table 1. Optimal ethical decision making requires open and timely communication between members of the pediatric team and the family, respecting their values, beliefs, and the fundamental principles of ethics. Parents may ethically and legally decide on behalf of children who are unable to express preferences, unless they are clearly acting against the child's best interest or are unable or unwilling to make such decisions. The wishes of a child who has obtained sufficient understanding and experience should be given significant consideration in the decision making process. Example, include ventilating advanced progressive muscular dystrophy patients. It is now widely accepted in bioethics that competent patient/family have the right to refuse treatment, even where that treatment may be life-saving or life-sustaining. The duty of care is not an absolute duty to preserve life by all means. There is no obligation to provide life sustaining treatment if the benefits of that treatment no longer outweigh the burden to the patient. It is never permissible to withdraw procedures designed to alleviate pain or promote comfort. For example, withholding hydration or antibiotics to treat transient infections is not justifiable. These infections may cause distress and pain, and treatment represents an important element of good palliative care.

Table 1: Fundamental ethical principles when considering DNR.

Duty of Care
1- Pediatric care has a primary intention of sustaining life and restoring health.
2- Whether or not the child can be restored to health, there is an absolute duty to comfort and to prevent pain and suffering.
Partnership of Care
1- The pediatric team and parents will enter a partnership of care, whose function is to serve the best interests of the child.
2- Children should be informed and listened to so that they can participate as fully as possible in decision making.
Legal Duty
1- Any treatment given with the intention of causing death is unlawful.
2- Children welfare is paramount and regard should be paid to their wishes.
3- Parents may make decisions on behalf of children provided that they act in their child's best interests.
4- There is no obligation to give treatment which is futile and burdensome.
5- Treatment goals may be changed in the case of children who are dying.
Respect for Children's Rights
1- Each child has the right for the highest standard of health care.
2- The child's right of freedom of expression and to receive information of all kinds should be respected.
3- A child who is capable of forming his/her view has the right to express those views freely in accordance with the age and maturity.
4- The families have the right to be given all necessary support in caring for their child and performing their child rearing responsibilities.

LEGAL ISSUES

An attempt to resuscitate the patient is considered futile in the absence of a reasonable potential of restoring vital functions. A physician is not legally obligated to make a specific diagnostic or therapeutic procedure available to a patient, even on specific request, if the use of such a procedure would be futile. However, it is important to recognize that there are some disagreements about how futility may be defined, about who defines futility, and about how judgments of futility are applied. The potential impact of this variability is highly significant given the recent evidence that perhaps as many as 88% of all DNR orders are based in part on the physician's judgment that resuscitation of the patient would be futile. On the other hand, if a physician wishes to continue treatment of a very ill child, but there is doubt about the benefit, the physician may be in a difficult legal position if the parents withhold consent. The physician should always act in the child's best interests not on his own believes as he will be ultimately responsible for his treatment decisions. Even in countries where ICU care is relatively well developed, considerable differences remain in physicians' attitudes toward end-of-life care. Therefore, the parents should always be participants in the care and decision making process. Older children should be involved to a degree appropriate for their age, experience and condition. For example, young children who have had several courses of chemotherapy or organ transplants will often have more informed views about further treatment than adult patients who are considering such treatment for the first time. It should be a duty of the professionals to assess the parent's and child's competency for decision making. Open and timely communication between the parents, patient, and the pediatric team is central to informed and ethical decision-making.

CLINICAL SETTING

In the labor room, neonates should almost always be resuscitated, particularly if there has been no prior discussion about DNR. Examples of clinical situations where DNR may be considered include: multiple congenital abnormalities that are incompatible with survival (*e.g.* anencephaly), gestational age of <23 weeks, and severe birth asphyxia with profound brain insult. Examples of conditions were DNR is considered in older children are summarized in Table **2**. They may include advanced anterior horn cell disease, severe head injury, advanced incurable malignancy, and brain death. Several studies have shown that children who die after a DNR decision are more likely to have chronic disease, in up to 80% of cases. The presence of chronic disease can have a significant impact on a parent's decision to limit treatment and on their ability to cope with that decision. One study showed that parents whose children had chronic disease were more likely to be satisfied with the care at end of life compared with parents whose children had suffered sudden or acute insults. These families may have had more time to reflect and accept the inevitability of their child's death.

Table 2: Common clinical situations where a DNR is considered.

Brain Death Absence of all brain and brainstem functions on neurological examination as a result of acute and irreversible brain insult. **Example:** Post cardiac arrest
Chronic Vegetative State A state of unawareness of self and environment in which the patient breathes spontaneously, has a stable circulation and shows cycles which simulates sleep and waking. The child in such a state is reliant on others for all care. **Example:** Post head injury, near drowning, hypoxic ischemic insult
"No Chance" Situation Treatment delays death but neither improves life's quality nor potential. Needlessly prolonging treatment in these circumstances is futile and burdensome and not in the best interests of the patient. **Example:** Ventilating advanced incurable neurodegenerative or metabolic disorder
"No Purpose" Situation The child may be able to survive with treatment, however, giving the treatment may not be in the child's best interest. The child may have a degree of irreversible impairment that it would be unreasonable to expect them to bear it. Continuing treatment might leave the child in a worse condition than already exists with the likelihood of further deterioration leading to poor quality of life. **Example:** Ventilating advanced progressive neuromuscular disorders
Unbearable Situation The child and/or family feel that further treatment is more than can be tolerated and they may wish to have treatment withheld or to refuse further treatment irrespective of the medical opinion that it may be of some benefit. **Example:** Palliative surgery or chemotherapy for advanced malignancy

CHILDREN WITH NEUROLOGICAL DISORDERS

One of the most challenging and difficult areas involves the question of withholding life sustaining treatment for children with severe neurological impairment. It is generally accepted to withhold life-prolonging treatment when the quality of life would be so afflicted as to be intolerable to the child. Examples include incurable progressive neurodegenerative or neurometabolic disorders (Table **2**). The quality of life could be considered intolerable when there is little prospect of meaningful awareness and interaction with others or the environment. The DNR decision is more difficult in patients with static (non-progressive) neurological disorders, such as severe cerebral palsy, as they may improve with time. Some of these children have an intolerable burden not only for themselves but also for their parents. Patients with less severe cerebral palsy are even more difficult to assess in regards to the acceptability of their disability. As well, some patients with severe impairment may have a life of good quality. Older children and adults may not view their residual disability as negatively as some normal people do, provided adequate support is available. Therefore, there must always be a commitment to the provision of high quality care for those with disability. Unfortunately, there are indications that such children have been discriminated against, for example when they compete for acute surgery. It is important to note that the condition of some of these patients may change with time and can be complicated by recurrent aspiration or chest infections. DNR can still be considered in those who require frequent ICU admission and ventilation as their quality of life deteriorates.

INITIAL ENCOUNTER

When it becomes evident that cure or acceptable quality of life is no longer possible or expected, the focus of care changes from prolonging life to ensuring a dignified death. In acute situations, such as those encountered in PICU, retrospective studies indicated that up to 60% of all deaths follow a DNR decision. The intensivist, who is often a stranger to the family, is frequently faced with the responsibility of writing the DNR. If such initial encounter occurs in the emergency room (ER), it is always necessary to give life-sustaining treatment first and then review the case. More experienced opinion and observation of the evolution of the clinical state in the light of investigations may further clarify the outcome, which may not be certain initially. All reversible causes for the child's condition must be excluded such as drugs and metabolic abnormalities. Many pediatricians and parents find the DNR decision psychologically and emotionally difficult. It may be easier for the parents to believe that everything possible has been done for their child. As well, some physicians may be reluctant to approach the subject of DNR with parents. Their reasons include, unfair to involve the parents in such decision, a DNR decision will not be accepted, or may cause a loss of trust. Religious and cultural issues often play a more vital role in decision making than economic considerations, especially in the Muslim communities. Discussions with the family about DNR should be conducted in a formal meeting. Meyer et al reported that up to 45% of parents had already considered the possibility of limiting therapy before discussing it with any staff member. This may reflect a shift from a more paternalistic medical attitude to a more family-centered care philosophy in pediatric institutions. Underlining the principles of autonomy and informed consent, the environment may allow families to be more confident in expressing their wishes and thoughts. Hence, families may already have a clear position about their opinion before a formal discussion takes place. Such discussions should including the nurses. This encourages a good physician-nurse relationship and strengthens the nature of the bedside relationship between nurses and families. Nurses normally engage in bedside discussion with parents about these issues long before there is an opportunity for the physicians to have the formal meeting. A USA study revealed a high rate of agreement between physicians and nurses on decision making and satisfaction with patients' treatment. The pediatric residents' presence in the formal meetings was poor and needs to be encouraged. Family conferences about end of life issues and DNR should be seen as an effective "teachable moment" for staff in training.

DECISION MAKING

Because of the difficulties in accurately predicting the outcome, patients may have a prolonged course in the PICU before a DNR decision is made. Direct neurologic involvement is frequently requested but not needed in all cases. A DNR consensus is achieved with some degree of difficulty in most cases. DNR decisions are more difficult in younger children, because one must rely on the best interests assessments of others, be they parents, pediatricians, or intensivists. A review of published literature on DNR decisions suggests that there is considerable practice variation around the world. In studies from North America and Europe, 30-65% of deaths in the PICU followed a DNR decision. The numbers may be significantly lower in developing or under developed countries. The differences in rate of active decision making could reflect either true differences in attitudes and clinical behavior with regard to the management of end of life, or alternatively may be due to different culture or resource-based PICU admission criteria whereby children with poor prognoses are not admitted. Lack of benefit from further therapy and expectation of imminent death is the main rationale for pediatric intensivists forgoing therapy. It is certainly different from quality of life and poor prognosis, both factors quoted by adult clinicians. In contrast, for parents, issues such as quality of life, likelihood of improvement, and perception of their child's pain are the predominant decision making factors. Pediatric intensivists may be more comfortable with the justification of lack of benefit and burden from additional therapy when death seems imminent. A survey among physicians and nurses with hypothetical case scenarios revealed that family preferences, probability of survival, and functional status are the major determinants influencing decisions about restricting life-support interventions in pediatrics, although there are markedly different attitudes depending on who is in charge of the patient. Various members of the medical team need to feel part of the decision making process depending on their knowledge, understanding and experience. Decisions should be made with the parents on the basis of knowledge and trust. Several studies found that parental involvement in the DNR decision making was common. However, physicians assume a more paternalistic role in some countries with little or no family consultation in the decision-making process. Studies from South America reported rates of family involvement in the decision-making process as low as 6%. In our Muslim communities, there is evidence that asking parents alone to be explicitly involved or take full responsibility for decisions involving life and death is not culturally or socially acceptable. Presence of extended family, and indirectly sounding out and taking into account their wishes, is more appropriate after assessing the resources and support services available. Ultimately, the clinical team carries the moral responsibility for decision making. There are different types and intensities of therapy that may be withheld, including cardiopulmonary resuscitation, mechanical ventilation, and intravenous inotropic agents. Antibiotics, nutrition and intravenous hydration need to continue to avoid discomfort and pain. Assisted feeding by nasogastric tube or gastrostomy should be considered in a child with a swallowing disorder due to a slowly progressive neurodegenerative disease. It is important to stress that some children go on to survive after a DNR decision. Treatment is withheld because it is futile but not with the intention to cause death (Table **3**).

Table 3: Summary of the guidelines for the use of DNR orders.

1- Efforts should be made to resuscitate patients except when circumstances indicate that CPR would be futile or not in best interests of the patient.
2- Physicians should discuss the possibility of arrest and encourages parents to express, in advance, their preferences regarding CPR. This should occur in an outpatient setting or soon during hospitalization, before the patient deteriorates.
3- In young children, a decision may be made by the parents in accordance with the patient's best interests.
4- If in the judgment of the treating physician, CPR would be futile, a DNR order may be entered into the patient's record with the basis for its implementation.
5- DNR orders only preclude resuscitative efforts in the event of arrest and should not influence other therapeutic and palliative interventions.
6- Hospital pediatric staffs should periodically review their experience, revise their DNR policies, and educate physicians regarding their role in decision-making.

EFFECTIVE COMMUNICATION

Talking to families about DNR is very challenging to most physicians. In one study, only 41% of the patients engaged in discussions with their physicians about CPR, and in 80% of the cases, physicians misunderstood the patient's preferences. Frequency of physician communication with families and the quality of information given keeps arising as a significant problem for relatives of dying patients in ICU, although in one pediatric survey 70% of parents believed that they were well informed. For full involvement, the parents must have adequate information and adequate time to understand and assess it, with time also to obtain alternate advice if they so wish. The final decision is made though the clinical team, which helps to alleviate the burden of guilt that some parents feel. A full record of communication with the family should be documented in the clinical record. Continuing communication and support maybe given by an involved social worker. As well, it is useful to include the primary pediatrician in the discussion, especially if they have known the family well. If they are not part of the ongoing discussion it is essential to keep them well informed of decisions and particularly of the child's death.

DIFFERENCE OF OPINION

The last days and hours of the child's life will most probably remain forever in the parents' minds and how their child dies is of critical importance for the parents' further lives. Because children are viewed as just beginning their lives one would likely infer that parents would display reluctance to agree to a DNR order than surrogates of older patients. Approximately half of the families in adult studies would agree with the DNR decision immediately or after only one meeting. Breen *et al.* reported conflict between staff and families in 48% of end-of-life discussion, and nearly 50% of families in another survey reported some form of conflict during their family member's stay in the adult ICU. A strong correlation was found with religious background. Even physicians, whose preferences' play a pivotal role in such decisions, may express diverse approaches to end-of-life decisions on the basis of their own religious background and country of origin. Within multicultural societies, understanding the patient's values and ethnocultural and religious traditions may improve end-of-life care by reducing the risk of conflicts and allowing more individualized care. In the Muslim society, this is not a major problem as most families have strong faith and believe that everything is in God's hands. The physician should make the important point of not trying to interfere with the death process once it starts. In most of our institutions, a favorable opinion of three physicians is needed for the approval of a DNR decision. However, when there is disagreement within the medical team or between the team and the family it is important to analyze its origins. It is possible that it reflects different understandings of the issues and that more time and better communication is needed.

However, unanimity on the part of the pediatric team is not essential. If there is anxiety about the degree of certainty behind the medical facts, further investigations could be considered. As well, resolving a difference of opinion between the team and the family is essential and may require a second opinion. Under these circumstances the family should still be fully supported by the team. Many major medical decisions require a second opinion for legal reasons as well as clinical assurance, such as brain death declaration. This could come from within the team, but if there is a more fundamental disagreement or erosion of trust, an expert opinion from outside the unit may be obtained. This could be organized by the consultant responsible for the care of the child. To secure greater confidence in the independence of the second opinion, the family may wish to arrange it themselves. The family should also be at liberty to change pediatrician and move to another consultant if this is possible. Input from religious advisors or other important sources of support to the family may be helpful. The hospital ethics committees may help in providing mediation and conciliatory functions. However, the legal and professional responsibility for decision making still rests with the consultant in charge of the case. In most cases, with effective communication and adequate time, the pediatric team and parents will come to agree.

SUPPORT AND BEREAVEMENT

The pending death of a child is one of the most devastating experiences that a parent can have and the quality of care at the end of life and after the child's death can have a major impact on the family's grieving. The family's presence at the bedside is an important element in the dying process. Although this is an emotionally charged situation, the family presence makes the process a clear and open one and conveys the shared nature of the decision. Each hospital should provide educational material both for staff and parents, taking into account the needs of different cultures. Many families will find their own support in different ways. In some situations families may prefer to care for their dying child at home. This may be when the focus of care becomes palliative and some period of time at home is anticipated. Careful communication and arrangements need to be made with home health care services. This will ensure that there is adequate support available and good continuity of care. Like the parents, health care providers will experience a wide range of emotions, both in the short term and over time. Work pressures can interfere with the resolution of these issues and failure to address them can lead to stress, lowered morale and divisions within the pediatric team. All involved staff need support, however, many may not know how to acknowledge or approach this need. Open discussions can be helpful and physicians should be encouraged to share their stresses and uncertainties with trainees and nurses. Additional support can be obtained from more senior staff, professional support workers, and religious scholars.

FUTURE PERSPECTIVES

Pediatric staff should have access to continuing education in DNR related ethics and communication. It has been recognized that in a scientifically based education it is essential that the psychological and spiritual dimensions of care are fully considered. Hospitals should have an educational clinical ethics forum that periodically meets to review difficult cases. Child bereavement organizations and parent support groups should be promoted and hence used in providing some of this training. The assessment of ethical issues, communication, knowledge and approaches should continue to form a mandatory part of the assessment of competence in clinical training. With limited available fund, offering expensive treatments and prolonged ICU care inevitably uses resources that may have been better used elsewhere. It is vital to conduct self-audit over the outcome in PICU and to obtain feedback from the involved families. As perspectives may change with time, such surveys should aim to be continuous. Research is needed in neurologically impaired children to determine what degree of disability is too burdensome. Undoubtedly, this is an area where it will be difficult to reach a consensus as the burden of disability depends on different perceptions.

SUMMARY

DNR should be considered when the continuation of intensive medical treatment is either futile or inflict unbearable suffering on the child. Physicians often feel that they have failed patients whose problems persist despite active treatment. However, in some circumstances, to continue life sustaining treatment is to offer care that is no longer in the child's best interest. Appropriate DNR decision depends on accurate knowledge of the child's condition and good relationships with the family. Conflicting emotions can affect the balance of both parental and professional judgment; however, good judgment will usually involve second opinions. The life of those with severe neurological disability is to be highly valued and they should be offered the best professional care. DNR decisions should never be hurried and there should always be respect for the child's life and a responsibility to relieve suffering.

BIBLIOGRAPHY

Jan MM. The decision of "do not resuscitate" in pediatric practice. Saudi Med J 2011;32(2):115-22.

CHAPTER 21

Brain Death Criteria

Abstract: Brain death implies the permanent absence of all cerebral and brainstem functions. The diagnosis of brain death is usually made clinically. The criteria require the occurrence of acute and irreversible CNS insult. Drug intoxication, poisoning, metabolic derangements, and hypothermia should be corrected for accurate brain death evaluation. At least two expert examiners are required to make the brain death determination. It is advisable to involve an independent examiner not involved in the patient's care or the recovery of donated organs. The objective of this chapter is to present updated guidelines for the process of brain death determination. All brain and brainstem functions should be absent on neurological examination including cerebral response to external stimuli and brain stem reflexes. An apnea test should be performed in all patients. However, if the clinical criteria cannot be applied, other confirmatory ancillary tests are required, particularly EEG and radionuclide scan. They are also needed to supplement the clinical assessment in young children. EEG is more reliable in the setting of hypotension or with disorders that lower intracranial pressure. While tests of brain blood flow are preferred in the setting of hypothermia, metabolic, or drug confounders.

Keywords: DNR, Resusitation, Brain death, Criteria, EEG, Isotope scan, Conciousness, Unresponsiveness, Vegetative, MRI, Ventillation.

BRAIN DEATH

Death is the irreversible cessation of all critical body functions. The brain is vital for integrating these critical body functions. Therefore, death of the brain is equivalent with whole body death. However, survival of other tissues or organs in isolation may continue beyond brain death. Brain death implies the permanent absence of all cerebral and brainstem functions. The term is specific and should not be used loosely to describe patients with severe brain damage or those in persistent vegetative states. Although specific details of diagnostic criteria vary in different countries, the fundamental definition of brain death has remained more or less the same. The diagnosis of brain death is highly related to organ donation. Most countries have specific brain death diagnostic mandates when applied to organ donation; however, general criteria are not always mandated. As well, most clinicians do not constantly adhere to the published guidelines. The variation of clinical practice is even greater in the pediatric field.

Table 1: Brain death criteria.

Etiology
• Established acute and irreversible CNS insult (*e.g.* trauma, hypoxia, ischemia)
• Exclude drug intoxication or poisoning that can be treatable or reversible
• Exclude other complicating or transient medical conditions that may affect the clinical assessment (severe electrolyte or acid-base disturbances)
Clinical Setting
• No hypothermia (temperature $\geq 36.5°C$)
• No hypotension (systolic blood pressure ≥ 90 mmHg)
• No sedation
• No neuromuscular paralysis
Clinical Examination
• Deep unresponsive coma
• No motor response, including response to pain stimulus above the neck
• No pupillary light reflex (midposition or dilated)
• No cough with tracheal suctioning
• No corneal or gag reflexes
• No oculovestibular reflexes (caloric response)
Apnea Testing
• No respiratory response ($PaCO_2 > 60$ mmHg or 20 mmHg more than baseline)

CLINICAL CRITERIA

The diagnosis of brain death is usually made clinically. The criteria require the presence of acute and irreversible CNS insult with absence of all brain and brainstem functions on neurological examination (Table 1). At least two expert examiners are required to make the brain death determination. The mandated number of examiners varies according to the country's law, ranging from 1-4. As well, some countries specifically require one of the physicians to be specialized in neurology. However, all examiners making the diagnosis of brain death should be familiar with the clinical criteria and comfortable in performing all aspects of the examination. It is advisable to involve an independent examiner not involved in the patient's care or the recovery of donated organs. Once the assessment is complete, a follow-up evaluation is mandatory in most, but not all, countries. The duration between the two assessments is age dependent (Table 2). It should be no less than 48-hours for infants 7 days to two months of age, 24 hours for those between two months to one year, and 12 hours for those between 1-18 years. An observation period for adults is optional in many countries, however, six hours is often recommended, particularly in the case of organ donation. A longer period of observation, up to 24 hours, is advisable in patients with potentially reversible hypoxic ischemic encephalopathy. In general, it is advisable to think of the process of brain death determination in four stages: etiology, clinical setting, examination, and apnea testing (Table 1).

Table 2: Differences between children and adults in the application of brain death criteria.

Criteria	Children	Adults
Age limit	Older than 7 postnatal days	Any age
Examination maneuvers	Oculocephalic reflex (doll's eye) Sucking reflex Rooting reflex	As in Table 1
Serial Examinations	Mandatory	Optional*
Interval between assessments	48 hours (Ages 7 days-2months) 24 hours (Ages 2 months-1 year) 12 hours (Ages 1-18 years)	6 hours
Ancillary tests	2 positive (7 days-2months) 1 positive (2 months-1 year) Optional after age 1 year**	Optional**

* Required if organ donation is considered or in hypoxic ischemic insult.

** Required only for clinical uncertainty or confounding factors.

CLINICAL CRITERIA

1- Etiology

Before starting the assessment, clinical or neuroimaging evidence of an acute and permanent CNS catastrophe that is compatible with the clinical diagnosis of brain death should be established. Trauma and hypoxic ischemic insult are the most common causes. However, any condition causing irreversible widespread brain injury can lead to brain death including infections or tumors. Complicating medical conditions that may confound the clinical assessment, such as severe electrolyte or acid-base disturbances, should be corrected for accurate evaluation. As well, potentially treatable or reversible drug intoxication or poisoning should also be excluded.

2- Clinical Setting

Normal body temperature and blood pressure are needed for accurate evaluation. Core temperature $\geq$36. 5° C, systolic blood pressure $\geq$90 mmHg, and normovolemic status are prerequisites. Hypothermia and hypotension may confound the diagnostic assessment of brain death; however, there is little evidence for a choice of threshold temperature. Therefore the 2006 Canadian forum recommendations substituted 34° C as a standard. The patient should also be off sedation or neuromuscular paralysis.

3- Clinical Examination

Adequate skills in performing the neurological examination are mandatory for proper assessment. The examination must demonstrate deep unresponsive coma with absent cerebral and brainstem functions including no motor response to pain stimulus above the neck, no pupillary light reflex (midposition or dilated), no corneal reflexes, no oculovestibular reflexes (caloric responses), no jaw jerk, no gag reflex, no cough with suctioning, and apnea as demonstrated by apnea test. In addition, oculocephalic (doll's eye maneuver), sucking, and rooting reflexes should be absent in children. The depth of coma must be assessed by documenting absent alerting response and no spontaneously or stimulus induced cortically originating movements. These include complex and purposeful movements, such as withdrawal or facial grimacing. Decerebrate and decorticate posturing are also originating from the brain and therefore should not be seen in brain death. Spontaneous, simple, non-purposeful movements originating from the spinal cord or peripheral nerve may occur in brain death. They are relatively common and may be triggered by tactile stimuli. They result from peripheral denervation or loss of cortical inhibitory input on lower motor neurons. Examples of these non-significant movements are listed in Table **3**. Finally, note that seizures are cortical in origin and therefore should not occur with brain death.

4- Apnea Testing

The apnea test is performed after all other criteria for brain death have been met. A positive apnea test demonstrates absence of respiratory response to a $PaCO_2$ >60 mmHg or 20 mmHg greater than baseline values. Simply disconnecting the ventilator is frequently associated with severe hypoxemia, bradycardia, and hypotension. These can be obviated by increasing inspired oxygen before and during the test. Preoxygenation eliminates respiratory nitrogen stores and accelerates oxygen transport. The fraction of inspired oxygen should be 1.0 for 10 minutes, up to a maximum PaO_2 of 200 mmHg. The patient is then disconnected from the ventilator. Oxygen is provided by a tracheal cannula at 6 L/minute. Visual observation for detecting respiratory movement should be carried out for 10 minutes. $PaCO_2$ should be remeasured just prior to reconnection to the ventilator to confirm that the target level was achieved. The test may need to be aborted because of hypotension or bradycardia. This may suggest inadequate preoxygenation, inadequate oxygenation during the test, or poor baseline cardiopulmonary status. Further confirmatory ancillary tests are necessary in this situation.

Table 3: Spinal cord or peripheral movements seen in brain death.

Facial twitches	Subtle, semi-rhythmic facial movements arising from the denervated facial nerve.
Finger twitching	Finger flexor movements.
Arm pronation	Upper limb pronation extension reflex.
Tonic neck reflexes "Lazarus sign"	Passive neck displacements, especially flexion, may be accompanied by complex truncal and extremity movements including adduction at the shoulders, flexion at the elbows, supination or pronation at the wrists, flexion of the trunk ("sitting up" type movements), and neck-abdominal muscle contraction or head turning to one side.
Truncal movements	Asymmetrical opisthotonic posturing of the trunk and preservation of superficial and deep abdominal reflexes.
Abnormal Babinski	Triple flexion response with flexion at the hip, knee, and ankle with foot stimulation.
Undulating toe sign	Alternating flexion-extension of the toes with passive displacement of the foot.

ANCILLARY TESTS

An accurate and comprehensive clinical examination is sufficient in determining brain death. Sometimes the clinical assessment cannot be accurate or complete. These situations include: when the cranial nerves cannot be adequately examined, when neuromuscular paralysis or sedation was used and is slow to clear due to multiorgan failure, and when the apnea test cannot be completed. In these situations, ancillary tests are necessary. Confirmatory ancillary testing is also required for infants less than one year. At least two positive tests are required routinely for infants less than two months of age and one positive test for those between 2 months to one year of age (Table **2**). Some countries mandate the routine use of a confirmatory test to supplement the clinical examination in older children and adults. In that case, such ancillary test should be highly suggestive of total and irreversible brain insult with no "false positives" results. Such a test should also be readily available, safe, and applied in all medical centers. Unfortunately, no currently available test for brain death meets all of these criteria. Studies examining their utility are limited with small biased samples limiting the detection of false-positive results. Individual tests have different strengths and weaknesses in different clinical settings, which may guide their selection. Ancillary tests used in confirming brain death are divided in two subgroups; neurophysiological and brain blood flow studies.

I- Clinical Neurophysiological Studies

Electroencephalography (EEG)

The EEG is the single most useful electrophysiological test of brain function. Electrocerebral silence (flat EEG) is expected in brain death. Technically, the EEG should contain no electrical cortical rhythms of >2 mV during a 30-minute recording. A specific EEG montage with long interelectrode distance and at least 18 channel recording is recommended. EEG is the most commonly ordered confirmatory test and is an essential part of the American criteria for the diagnosis of brain death in young children. However, note that the EEG summates synaptic potentials from the cerebral neocortex and does not reveal potentials from subcortical structures, such as the brain stem or thalamus. Therefore, the EEG may be flat or isoelectric in the presence of viable neurons in the brain stem. The EEG is also vulnerable to confounders, and may be isoelectric in cases of sedation, hypothermia, or metabolic disturbances. In these cases, a flat EEG recording is falsely positive. In addition, electrical artifacts are frequently recorded, especially in the intensive care unit. Artifacts may be mistaken by the less experienced interpreter for residual cortical activity.

Evoked Potentials

Somatosensory evoked potentials (SSEPs) and brainstem auditory evoked potentials (BAEPs) are used infrequently as ancillary tests. In SSEPs, the bilateral absence of the parietal sensory cortex responses (N19-P22) in response to median nerve stimulation is supportive of brain death. The absence of brainstem responses to an auditory stimulus (Waves III to V) in the presence of preserved cochlear response (Wave I) is required for a BAEP result to support the diagnosis of brain death. These tests activate discrete and restricted sensory pathways in the brainstem. Therefore, they do not test the functional integrity of other CNS structures. As well, peripheral lesions outside the CNS may affect their results. Falsely positive results, particularly in patients with primary brainstem pathology, have been reported. However, components of SSEPs and BAEPs are minimally affected by sedative drugs and anesthetics.

II- Brain Blood Flow Studies

Tests demonstrating absent blood flow to the brain are generally considered confirmatory of whole brain death. Brain death is usually associated with increased intracranial pressure (ICP) due to tissue edema or mass effects. Lack of cerebral blood flow occurs when the ICP exceeds the systemic arterial pressure flow. Tests of cerebral blood flow include nuclear medicine, cerebral angiography, transcranial Doppler, magnetic resonance angiography (MRA), and computed tomographic angiography (CTA). These tests are not confounded by drugs, metabolic disorders, or hypothermia. However, the systemic blood pressure should be adequate. The presence of some arterial blood flow in the intracranial compartment does not always preclude the diagnosis of brain death. This may occur if the intracranial pressure is lowered, such as in patients with skull fractures, craniotomy, ventricular drain, or in infants with open cranial sutures. Acknowledging the existing limitations of these tests, further research validating current and evolving techniques of brain blood flow imaging are needed.

Nuclear Medicine

The two main radionuclide techniques used in the evaluation of brain death are radionuclide angiography with nonlipophillic agents and parenchymal imaging using lipophilic agents. The most commonly used radionuclide tracer is 99mTc-labeled hexamethylpropyleneaminoxime (HMPAO). The tracer penetrates into the brain parenchyma in proportion to regional blood flow and shows no significant redistribution for several hours, making it easy to perform and interpret the images. The absence of isotope uptake ("hollow skull phenomenon") indicates no brain perfusion and supports the diagnosis of brain death. The test is useful in pediatric patients with limited false-positive and false-negative results.

Cerebral Angiography

Traditional 4-vessel cerebral angiography is the "gold standard" among cerebral blood flow tests for brain death. However, the test is invasive and requires transportation to the radiology department. Cerebral angiography usually demonstrates absent blood flow beyond the carotid bifurcation or Circle of Willis. Contrast stasis or delayed filling in intracranial arteries is an earlier stage preceding absent filling. False-negative result showing some normal blood flow in some intracranial vessels may occur rarely with lowered intracranial pressure (*e.g.* craniotomy, VP shunts, or infants with open sutures). Therefore, cerebral angiography is not only invasive, but also risky, and may be inaccurate.

Transcranial Doppler (TCD)

Transcranial Doppler (TCD) is an innovative, safe, and noninvasive tool for the bedside monitoring of static and dynamic cerebral blood flow. Small systolic peaks without diastolic flow or a reverberating flow pattern suggest high vascular resistance and support the diagnosis of brain death. Temporal bone thickening precludes the evaluation in up to 25% of patients. This and other technical limitations may give false positive results and therefore limit the value of TCD. Inspite of the currently reported sensitivity of 70% and specificity of 97%, the procedure requires further study, particularly in young children.

Magnetic Resonance Angiography (MRA)

Absence of arterial blood flow on MRA supports the diagnosis of brain death. Small case series suggest that it may be a useful test in brain death. MRA is problematic in unstable patients as the patient is required to lie flat for long time. There are also practical difficulties in performing close clinical monitoring of these unstable patients. MRA may prove more useful in the future.

Computed Tomographic Angiography (CTA)

CTA and CT perfusion are more invasive than MRA requiring contrast injection. Several case reports document findings of absent cerebral circulation perfusion in patients with brain death. The test needs further study before further recommendation.

Misdiagnoses

Rarely, brain death can be misdiagnosed if the previously described protocol was not followed, particularly by less experienced physicians. Hypothermia, drug intoxication, and metabolic encephalopathy can present with severe brain and brainstem dysfunction simulating brain death. Therefore, they should be corrected before such declaration is made. Occasionally, locked-in syndrome and severe Guillain-Barré syndrome may produce a neurological examination consistent with brain death. The locked-in syndrome is a consequence of focal insult to the base of the pons, usually by embolic occlusion of the basilar artery. Consciousness is preserved; however, the patient cannot move the limbs, trunk, or face. Only voluntary blinking and vertical eye movements remain intact. Patients with this syndrome have been mistakenly believed to be unconscious. Patients with primary brainstem pathology who are believed to be brain dead should be carefully examined to ensure that they are not locked-in. Detailed history taking and careful neurological examination will easily exclude Guillain-Barré syndrome. All potential brain death mimics should not be mistaken for brain death if the clinical brain death criteria are applied.

Communicating the News

Once the diagnosis of brain death is confirmed, such information should be communicated to the family and relatives. Communicating such news is often both difficult and emotionally unwelcome (see chapter 22). Most physicians do not feel comfortable in such difficult situations. At the same time, it is important that the transfer of such information is done well as the manner in which bad news is conveyed to relatives can significantly influence their emotions, beliefs, and attitudes towards the medical staff, and the future. Most families find the attitude of the news giver, combined with the clarity of the message and the news giver's knowledge to answer questions as the most important aspects of giving such bad news. Note that the perception that death has occurred differs from one person to another. The diagnosis of brain death is intricately linked to the issue of organ donation and may influence family member's decision making. Bereaved family members approached to donate the organs of their brain dead relative should have a good understanding of what this diagnosis means. The reliability and differences between cardio-pulmonary *versus* brain based criteria of death should be explained. In many developed countries, people can decide on whether they will be donors upon getting their driver license. This will ease the pressure on their relatives who may have difficulty accepting the responsibility of making such decision at the time of death. From a parent's perspective, brain death and organ donation are neither morally or medically straightforward concepts. There is clearly a strong need for more research and clinical training in communication issues regarding brain death and end-of-life care with families in critical care situations.

Prognosis

Brain death rarely lasts for more than few days before it is followed by whole body death. Brain ischemia leads to sympathetic nervous system collapse with vasodilatation and cardiac dysfunction. Pulmonary edema and diabetes insipidus are common early consequences of brain death and may precipitate cardiopulmonary failure. Rare cases of prolonged somatic survival of clinically brain dead adults have been reported. However, the diagnosis of brain death becomes doubtful in the face of prolonged clinical stability, particularly in pediatric patients. Some families have religious beliefs that oppose the equivalence of brain death with death. In Saudi Arabia, a religious law (Islamic Fatwa) allows physicians to discontinue life support over the family's objection in patients with documented brain death. However, decision delay, further education, support, and negotiation are advocated in such situations. The potential for organ donation may offer comfort to some bereaved families, however, it should not be the impetus for the diagnosis of brain death.

SUMMARY

Brain death is the complete and irreversible loss of cerebral and brain stem functions. It is considered to be equivalent to whole body death. The diagnosis of brain death is usually made clinically; however, certain prerequisites are needed. These include an established acute and permanent cause, and exclusion of drug intoxication, poisoning, metabolic derangements, and hypothermia. The neurological examination must demonstrate deep unresponsive coma, no cerebral response to external stimuli, and absent brain stem reflexes. An apnea test should be performed in all patients meeting all other brain death criteria. Confirmatory ancillary tests are required when the clinical criteria cannot be applied and to supplement the clinical assessment in young children. EEG and radionuclide scan are the two most commonly used tests for brain death confirmation. EEG is more reliable in the setting of hypotension, craniotomies, or other factors that lower intracranial pressure. While tests of brain blood flow are preferred in the setting of hypothermia and metabolic or drug confounders.

BIBLIOGRAPHY

Jan MM: Brain Death Criteria: The Neurological Determination of Death. Neurosciences 2008;13(4):350-5.

CHAPTER 22

Communicating Bad News

Abstract: Many traumatic, infectious, vascular, and neoplastic neurological disorders carry poor prognoses for complete neurological recovery. These disorders may result in chronic disability with multiple medical and neurological complications. The common practice of consanguineous marriage in Saudi Arabia results in a high prevalence of many inherited and genetic neurological and metabolic disorders. Many of these children exhibit progressive deterioration in cognitive, language, and/or motor function. Because of the high incidence of such disorders, many of which cannot be characterized, the necessity of facing parents with discussions regarding prognosis is not uncommon.

Keywords: Communication, Giving, Bad, Neurological, News, DNR, Resusitation, Brain death, Unresponsiveness, Vegetative, Ventillation.

INTRODUCTION

Informing parents of the diagnosis of a chronic illness or disability in their child is a difficult task. At the same time, it is important that the informing is done well. How parents are told can significantly influence their emotions, beliefs, and their attitudes towards the child, medical staff, and future. Most families describe shock, the state of being upset and subsequent depression after hearing the news of a bad neurological disorder such as Neurofibromatosis. However, the attitude of the news giver, combined with the clarity of the message and the knowledge in providing answers to questions have been found to be important aspects of giving bad news. Most physicians are not well prepared to deal with communicating bad news as in their training they usually receive little or no formal education regarding the process. While most young physicians wanted instructions on how to break bad news, yet only 45% had received any such instruction. Additionally it is accepted that many physicians are unaware of their difficulties in giving information in a clear and comprehensive way. This chapter attempts to provide general guidelines regarding the process of communicating neurological bad news to parents. Nearly all senior physicians are aware that communicating details of unfortunate, especially chronic or progressively deteriorating, neurological conditions to parents become easier and less emotionally distasteful with increased experience. It is the objective of this chapter to attempt to capture such experience and articulate it in such a way that the younger clinicians can be the beneficiaries – at least to the point that the wheel does not need to be completely rediscovered by each individual facing the responsibility in early practice.

PREPARATION FOR BREAKING THE BAD NEWS

Physicians must prepare adequately for the process of communicating bad news. This process is not only stressful to parents, but also to most physicians. The ideal would be that all physicians take an educational course that deals with breaking bad news. Several studies have documented that such educational programs provided to medical students, residents, or other physicians, improves their ability to council and inform parents. In one study, formal instructions improved the humanistic skills of the provider as they relate to the delivery of bad news. As well, most students involved in one program found it enjoyable, useful, and found that it increased their sense of competence and their ability to formulate a strategy for such situations. An educational program should teach the physician various methods of managing stress and crises intervention. The education should involve clarification of personal attitudes, discussion of previous personal encounters of the participants, examination of various communication modalities, analyses of different methods of addressing and understanding parents' feelings and emotions, and exposure to various coping skills in dealing with the emotions of the one breaking the bad news. If a formal educational program is not available to the physician, self-education and learning from the literature and sharing the experience of more senior physicians in the field can be helpful. Physicians must realize what impact the news can have on the parents, must overcome the potential fear of being blamed for the message, and must not accept a sense of failure for not being able to remedy or improve the natural history of a bad diagnosis.

Mohammed M. S. Jan

PREPARATION FOR THE INITIAL INTERVIEW

The key for good communication is to carefully prepare for the initial interview. Adequate time must exist so that the meeting is not rushed. At least 30, and preferably 60, minutes should be reserved. The physician should know the child very well and should have at her/his fingertips all relevant medical facts. Detailed discussions with the other members of the team and consultants who evaluated the child are needed as part of the interview. The diagnosis should be adequately documented and pending results and their possible implications and any suspicions should be outlined. Reaching a specific diagnosis is of clear importance for providing appropriate therapy, prognosis, and genetic counseling. CT and MRI images could be used to illustrate any structural central nervous system abnormalities.

It is always helpful to find out how much the parents know or suspect before the meeting. Awareness of the family's dynamics and their socio-cultural expectations would further facilitate the physician's role and interactions during the initial interview. Arrangements should be made with both parents to attend the meeting. The common practice in our culture of telling the father first and giving him the task of breaking the bad news to the family should probably be discouraged. Studies have documented that when parents are told together they derive support from each other. In this way, each parent will receive first hand information, will more likely remember what has been said, and will have a chance to ask questions. The presence of other extended relatives should be discouraged, at least in the initial instance. Certainly, there are often important support persons who, by virtue of their relationship to the family, their stations in life, or their background education, the families may wish to have present at subsequent interviews. This is understandable and acceptable; however, it is our practice not to allow more than three family members in such meetings. It is optional to have the child present during the interview. We usually allow infants and younger children to attend, but discourage older children who may become unnecessarily exposed to poorly understood details and to their parent's emotional reactions.

When, Where, and Who Should Break the Bad News?

The neurological bad news should be communicated to the parents as soon as possible after medical investigation is confirmative and preferably before the child is discharged from hospital. The news should be given in person and never over the telephone. A comfortable meeting room to provide privacy in a friendly atmosphere is ideal. Preferably the room should be away from the clinic or ward area to avoid distractions and allow no interruption. The consultant who knows the child best and is closest to the family is the one who should break the news. This is usually the pediatric neurologist or neurosurgeon. However, as alluded to earlier, if the family has a regular family physician in whom they have obvious confidence; it may be beneficial to have her/him participate in the interview. Selected members of the team may attend this meeting including the intern, resident, nurse, social worker, and other involved sub-specialists. In order not to overwhelm the parents, we usually prefer the attendance of a maximum of four team members who know the child and the family best. All such members should have had good interactions with, and are well known to, the family. One consultant should lead the interview and direct the discussion in order to provide consistency and continuity. Only in very exceptional circumstances should interns, residents, or nurses communicate neurological bad news. Residents show a general lack of competence in delivering bad news, particularly relating to the elicitation of the parent's perspectives, *i.e.* they lacked a patient centered interviewing style. This is perhaps predictable, given their limited experience, which, of course, improves with increased training. In fact, we always encourage the junior members to attend these meetings as part of their learning experience.

How to Break Neurological Bad News?

All parents are anxious during the initial interview, as more times than not they have some inkling that they are about to receive difficult-to-accept information about their child. The physician must exhibit maturity, friendliness, and firmness on the background of respect and trust. The literature would support the notion that most parents prefer communication of information and feelings by a physician who clearly possesses a deportment of confidence. Sharp and colleagues considered that their strongest preferences were for physicians to show caring, to allow parents to talk, and to allow parents to show their own feelings. The lead physician needs to introduce the members of the team attending the meeting. We always allow the parents to tell us what they already know about the child's condition and how they think he or she is doing. We frequently begin by saying, "what is your understanding of … [your child's]… condition". This may ease their initial excessive anxiety, improve the interaction, and make the process easier as most parents have a good sense of the seriousness of their child's condition, as already noted. Further, and probably most importantly, it provides the best entrance into the discussion and there is no doubt about the fact that the most difficult part of such an interview is its initiation.

It is best if the information is given in small but balanced amounts. Giving the information in stages is better than presenting the parents with all the information at once. Start with general medical issues and then proceed to more difficult and specific prognostic information. The information should include the diagnosis, cause, features, complications, treatments, and prognosis. During the communication of the bad news, the provider should be open, frank, honest, and should maintain good eye contact. Explanations should be kept simple, direct, and at a level of understanding that is both clear to the parents and keep to a minimum any reference to medical jargon. However, the informational content and medical details can be expressed differently according to the parent's educational level. In this time era, many parents are knowledgeable and can handle complex medical information, particularly with the advent of the Internet resources.

Throughout the discussion, the balance between avoiding pessimism, providing hope, and being realistic needs to be maintained. Pointing out the child's strengths and weaknesses without false reassurance is needed. It is important to point out the remarkable ability of the developing central nervous system to adapt and recover following insults. It is important to emphasize that this "plasticity" of the brain can facilitate continuing recovery for several months to a year following any insult to the nervous system, *e.g.* such as in the case of trauma, vascular compromise, etc. We usually simplify this concept by stating that the undamaged areas of the brain can take over some of the functions of the damaged areas, as a means of emphasizing the concept of plasticity. Avoid overstating the possible improvements to prevent false hope of complete neurological recovery. Some parents have strong religious beliefs. Recognizing and understanding when strong religious faith prevails can be of immeasurable benefit with the appropriately placed emphasis. In Saudi Arabia for example, Moslems have faith in God and in life after death. Part of this faith is the acceptance that God's will is inevitable and the exact future is in his hands. This belief gives the parents internal satisfaction and happiness with the child's outcome as long as they are confident not only in their faith but also in the medical team. Humor during the interview should be avoided because of possible misinterpretation by anxious parents. Sensitivity to both informational content and parents' responses and emotional reactions is critical. When bad news is broken insensitively, the impact can be distressing for both giver and recipient. For the recipient, especially, the effect can be long lasting. Years later, parents will continue to remember exactly who and how the bad news was conveyed. Allow both parents to ask questions, but maintain the direction of the discussion. Avoid discussing hypothetical questions or scenarios, and promise the parents that problems and new issues will be discussed when they arise. We usually tell parents that more time is needed to clarify the course of each child's disease and we cannot always predict the future accurately. Avoid arguing with the parents and try your best to be both empathetic and supportive of their emotional responses. At some point during the final part of the discussion we usually indicate something like "We would rather not be in this position of having to confront you with this news, but this is where we are now, and this is the point from which we must proceed". Assure them that there will be future meetings, more than one if necessary, to discuss the child's problems in more detail and answer any new questions which might arise. Advise the parents to write a list of questions that they may have in the near future for the next meeting. At the end of the interview, the physician should leave and give the parents time together in the room. This is especially important after the initial interview.

Repeated Interviews

Sequential interviews usually are best conducted by the same provider for continuity of care and consistency of the given message. Again, the parents must be allowed to update you with the child's condition. Confidence in their ability to cope with and manage the child must be conveyed to them. The information given in the first meeting should be summarized and then expanded, updated and further questions answered. One must make certain that the parents understood what was said in the initial meeting in terms of their interpretation of the implications assigned to the diagnosis. Some times an anxious parent may misunderstand the information or miss some important components. Important points should be stressed by repeating them in different ways. Parents' question lists can be answered and new diagnostic and therapeutic issues can be addressed. At this stage, genetic counseling, where appropriate, may have been provided to the family. If it has not been raised, it should be briefly discussed. Concentrate on positive aspects of the management including the appropriate involvement of a multidisciplinary team including physiotherapy, occupational therapy, nutritionist, and those involved in Developmental Medicine. The parents must be assured that additional equipment to assist the child's disabilities, where appropriate, can be provided, *e.g.* wheelchair, glasses, hearing aids, etc, as well as medications to treat any complications, *e.g.* sleep disorders, epilepsy, spasticity, etc. The effects of these treatments should be clearly stated as being symptomatic and not curative, in order to prevent false hope of complete neurological recovery.

Further Support

The parents should receive adequate medical, social, and emotional support. Involvement of other sub-specialists as they relate to each specific case (*e.g.* endocrine, metabolic or genetic consultants, etc) is important to assure the parents of the adequacy of medical care. Physicians should be open to the concept of a second opinion. When brought up by parents, the physician must not convey the outward appearance of being irritated or personally offended. Many times this idea is brought up under social pressure. The physician should facilitate this process. This facilitation, especially if it is presented as a very welcomed suggestion, will greatly relieve bereaved parents and increase their confidence in you, as the treating consultant. One should attempt to help the family and direct them to the right person who can provide a reliable second opinion. Physicians should also keep a list and have contacts with various local disability foundations and service associations that could benefit the parents and the child. Social support should also be encouraged with the coordination of the case social worker. Parents should be encouraged to show and share their feelings with close family members and friends to strengthen their support group. In the Saudi Arabian society, there is a tendency to keep these issues secret even from the closest family members and friends. Our suggestion is that such issues should be discussed with the family and the parents should be encouraged to contact family support groups. If these are not available, telephone numbers of families with similarly affected children (after obtaining their consent) would be helpful as most parents desire parent-to-parent referral. The potential powerful positive effect of this latter strategy cannot be over-emphasized. In Saudi Arabia, most parents also benefit from religious and spiritual support with readings from the holy book and discussions with eligible scholars.

SUMMARY

This chapter reviewed and detailed an outline regarding the process of communicating neurological bad news to parents. In summary, physicians must prepare adequately for this process. The skills necessary for breaking bad news well can be acquired through organized undergraduate and postgraduate education, which emphasizes a good working doctor-parent relationship. Neurological bad news should be communicated to both parents as early as possible. Parents prefer the physicians who show a genuine caring attitude, who encourage and allow them to talk, and who show understanding of their emotional responses. The balance between avoiding pessimism, providing hope, and being realistic needs to be maintained throughout the interview. Sensitivity to both informational content and parents' responses and emotional reactions is critical. Subsequent meetings should be arranged to stress important points, update, and answer their ongoing, and indeed often recurrent, questions. Confidence should be conveyed in the parents' ability to cope with and manage the child.

In twenty-first century medicine this part of the "art" of medicine is too often sacrificed in deference to the science of medicine. Such a sacrifice not only contravenes the oath which we all take upon graduation from a Faculty of Medicine but indeed germinates much of the criticism which seems to have arisen towards physicians over the past two or three decades. Many physicians may already follow some of the proposed guidelines. However, hopefully the details, as outlined in the foregoing, will assist practitioners in communicating neurological bad news to parents more effectively and compassionately.

BIBLIOGRAPHY

Jan MMS, Girvin JP: The Communication of Neurological Bad News to Parents. Can J Neurol Sci 2002;29:78-82.

Index

A
Abducent nerve, 10
Absence epilepsy, 48,49,54
Acidemia, 43
ADEM, 113
Adenoma sebaceum, 8
Adrenoleukodystrophy, 39
Alexander disease, 35
Alpers disease, 59
Amblyobia, 30
Aminoaciduria, 43
Ammonia, 43
Anterior fontanels, 7
Anterior horn cell, 84
Anticonvulsants, 56
Apneustic breathing, 7
Apraxia, 13
Arterial thromboembolism, 90
Asphyxia, 28
Ataxia telangiectasia, 99
Ataxia, 98
Ataxic breathing, 7
Athetosis, 27, 96
Attention deficit, 37
Audiometry, 30
Aura, 63
Autism, 37

B
Baclofen, 32
Bad news, 129
Basal ganglia, 27
Bell's palsy, 10
Benzodiazepines, 56,59
Bilirubin, 28
Blindness, 30
Botulinum toxin, 32
Brain death, 123
Breath holding spells, 51
Bulbar palsy, 29

C
Café au lait spots, 8
Calcification, 54
Calcium channels, 56
Canavan disease, 35
Carbamazepine, 56
Carbidopa, 94
Carnitine, 45
Central core disease, 88

Centronuclear, 88
Cerebellar ataxia, 12
Cerebral edema, 8
Cerebral infarction, 90
Cerebral palsy, 27
Cherry red spot, 38
Cheyne Stokes, 7
Chorea, 27
Choreoathetosis, 27
Chromosomes, 21
Clonazepam, 56
Coenzyme Q, 45
Coma, 8
Consciousness, 8
Corpus callosum, 23
Corticosteroids, 114
Cranial nerves, 9
Craniosynostosis, 7

D
Deafness, 30
Decerebrate posturing, 11
Decorticate posturing, 11
Demyelination, 111
Developmental delay, 21
Devic syndrome, 112
Diazepam, 56, 59, 75
Diplegia, 28
Diplopia, 10
DNR, 116
Dopa responsive, 94
Double hemiplegia, 28
Duchenne dystrophy, 88
Dysmorphism, 8
Dyspepsia, 51
Dystonia, 94
Dystrophy, 88

E
Edema, 8
Edrophonium, 89
EEG, 36, 53, 74
EMG, 12, 36
Encephalitis, 78
Encephalomyelitis, 113
Epilepsia partialis continua, 59
Epilepsy, 47, 62
Ethosuximide, 56
Extraocular movements, 10

F
Facial nerve, 10

Fainting, 51
Fasciculations, 12
Feeding problems, 29
Fibrillations, 12
Fontanels, 7
Fosphenytoin, 56
Fragile X syndrome, 22
Frontal lobe epilepsy, 65, 68

G
Gabapentin, 56
Gait, 98
Gangliosidosis, 38
Gigantism, 7
Glasgow Coma Scale, 8
Glutaric acidemia, 43
Gower sign, 11
Growth, 7
Guillain Barre, 87

H
Hallervorden Spatz, 36
Head circumference, 7
Headache, 105
Hearing loss, 30
Hemiplegia, 28, 90
Hemispherectomy, 60
Hepatotoxicity, 59
Herniation, 109
Hirsutism, 57
Hydrocephalus, 109
Hyperammonemia, 43, 44
Hyperexplexia, 50
Hypothyroidism, 23
Hypotonia, 83
Hypoxia, 13
Hypsarrhythmia, 53

I
Infarction, 90
Inferior oblique, 10
Inferior rectus, 10
Intracranial pressure, 109
Intravenous IG, 89, 103
Ion channels, 57
Isovaleric acidemia, 43

J
Jerks, 48, 49
Jitteriness, 50
Juvenile myoclonic, 55

K

Karyotyping, 22, 23
Kayser Fleischer ring, 38
Keppra, 56
Kernicterus, 28
Kernig sign, 8
Ketogenic diet, 60
Krabbe disease, 35, 39

L

Lactate, 43
Lactic acidosis, 43
Lafora body, 35
Lamotrigine, 56
Language delay, 24
Lead poisoning, 24
Lennox Gastaut syndrome, 55
Leukodystrophy, 39
Levetiracetam, 56
Levodopa, 94
Lisch nodule, 38
Lorazepam, 56, 59
Lumbar puncture, 74
Lysosomal disorders, 35

M

Macrocephaly, 7
Magnetic resonance, 54, 74
Marcus gun pupil, 9
Megalencephaly, 7
MELAS, 92
Meningitis, 79
Mental retardation, 24, 28
Metabolic acidosis, 43
Metabolic disorders, 42
Metachromatic, 35
Methylmalonic acidemia, 43
Microcephaly, 7
Midazolam, 59
Migraine, 105
Mitochondrial disorders, 39
Motor examination, 11
Movement disorders, 94
Multiple sclerosis, 111
Muscular dystrophy, 88
Myasthenia gravis, 89
Myoclonic epilepsy, 48
Myopathy, 88

N

Neck stiffness, 8
Nerve conduction, 36

Neurocutaneous syndromes, 8
Neurofibromatosis, 8
Neurological exam, 6, 14
Neurological history, 3
Neurontin, 56
Neuropathy, 36
Niemann Pick disease, 38
Night terrors, 51
Nitrazepam, 56
Nonepileptic, 50, 51
Nystagmus, 38

O
Obesity, 7
Oculomotor nerve, 10
Oligoclonal bands, 112
Optic nerve, 9
Organic academia, 43

P
Palate, 10
Palmar grasp, 12
Pancreatitis, 28
Papilledema, 9
Parachute reflex, 12
Paraldehyde, 59
Paraplegia, 28
Parkinson disease, 10
Partial seizures, 48, 63
Partial status epilepticus, 59
Pelzaeus Merzbacher, 35
Periventricular, 28, 31
Petit mal epilepsy, 54
Phenobarbitone, 56
Phenytoin, 56
Photophobia, 106
Plantar grasp, 12
Port wine stain, 8
Position sense, 13
Prematurity, 28
Primidone, 56
Pseudoseizures, 51
Ptosis, 10
Pupilary reflex, 10
Pyridoxine, 42

Q
Quadriceps, 11
Quadriplegia, 28

R
Reflexes, 11

Retardation, 24, 28
Rett syndrome, 22
Rheumatic fever, 96
Rigidity, 27, 94
Rolandic epilepsy, 55
Romberg test, 13
Rooting reflex, 12, 19
Roseola, 72

S
Sabril, 56
Scoliosis, 7
Segawa disease, 94
Seizures, 47, 62, 72
Sensory ataxia, 102
Shagreen patch, 8
Short stature, 7
Shuddering attack, 50
Sickle cell anemia, 92
Simple partial seizure, 48, 63
Skin examination, 7
Skull examination, 7
Sleep myoclonus, 50
Sleep wake cycle, 29
Snellen chart, 9
Sodium benzoate, 40
Sotos syndrome, 7
Spastic diplegia, 28
Spastic hemiplegia, 28
Spastic quadriplegia, 28
Spasticity, 32
Speech delay, 24
Spikes, 53
Spinal dysraphism, 8
Spinal muscular atrophy, 84
Static encephalopathy, 21
Status epilepticus, 59
Steroids, 114
Stevens Johnson, 57
Strabismus, 30
Stroke, 90
Stereognosis, 13
Sturge Weber, 8
Sucking reflex, 12
Sydenham chorea, 96

T
Tandom MS, 38
Tegretol, 56
Telengiectasia, 99
Tendon reflexes, 11
Tension headache, 105
Thiamine, 45

Thiopental, 59
Thromboembolism, 90
Todd paralysis, 65
Tonic neck reflex, 12
Topiramate, 56
Tourette syndrome, 51
Tremor, 96
Triceps reflex, 11
Trochlear nerve, 10
Tuberous sclerosis, 8

U
Urea cycle defects, 44

V
Vagus nerve, 10
Valproic acid, 56
VEP, 36
Vigabatrin, 56
Visual acuity, 9
Visual aura, 63
VN stimulation, 60

W
Weakness, 87
White matter, 36

X
X-linked disorders, 35